plant

magic

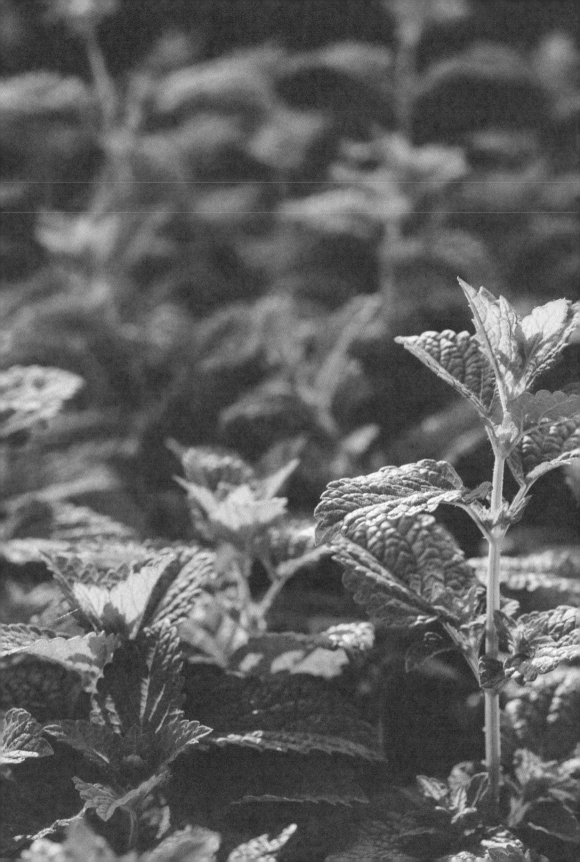

plant magic

HERBALISM IN REAL LIFE

CHRISTINE BUCKLEY

ROOST BOOKS

Roost Books
An imprint of Shambhala Publications, Inc.
4720 Walnut Street
Boulder, Colorado 80301
roostbooks.com

Disclaimer: Eating wild plants may be risky due to the nature of look-alike poisonous plants. The information presented here is thorough and accurate to the best of our knowledge, but it is essential that you always practice extreme caution and use your best judgment when foraging. Please do not attempt self-treatment of a medical problem without consulting a qualified health practitioner. Shambhala Publications and the author disclaim any and all liability in connection to the collection and consumption of wild plants and the use of the instructions in this book.

9 8 7 6 5 4 3 2 1

First Edition
Printed in China

⊗This edition is printed on acid-free paper that meets the American National Standards Institute Z39.48 Standard.
♻Shambhala Publications makes every effort to print on postconsumer recycled paper. For more information please visit www.shambhala.com.

Roost Books is distributed worldwide by Penguin Random House, Inc., and its subsidiaries.

Designed by Lizzie Allen

Library of Congress Cataloging-in-Publication Data
Names: Buckley, Christine, 1983– author.
Title: Plant magic: herbalism in real life / Christine Buckley.
Description: First edition. I Boulder: Roost Books, [2020] I Includes bibliographical references and index.
Identifiers: LCCN 2019007007 j ISBN 9781611806557 (pbk.: alk. paper)
Subjects: LCSH: Herbs—Therapeutic use. I Holistic medicine.
Classification: LCC RM666.H33 B832 2020 I DDC 615.3/21—dc23
LC record available at https://lccn.loc.gov/2019007007

For Kumajiro and the trees.

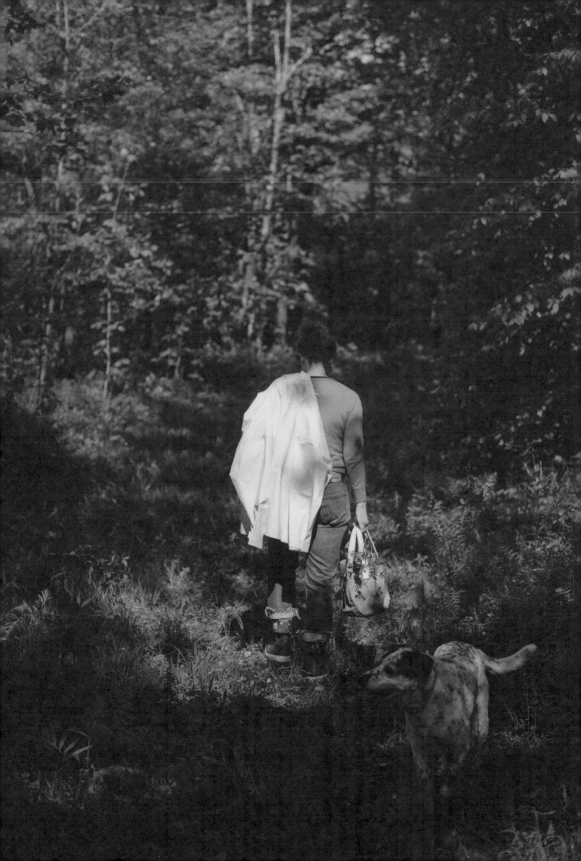

Contents

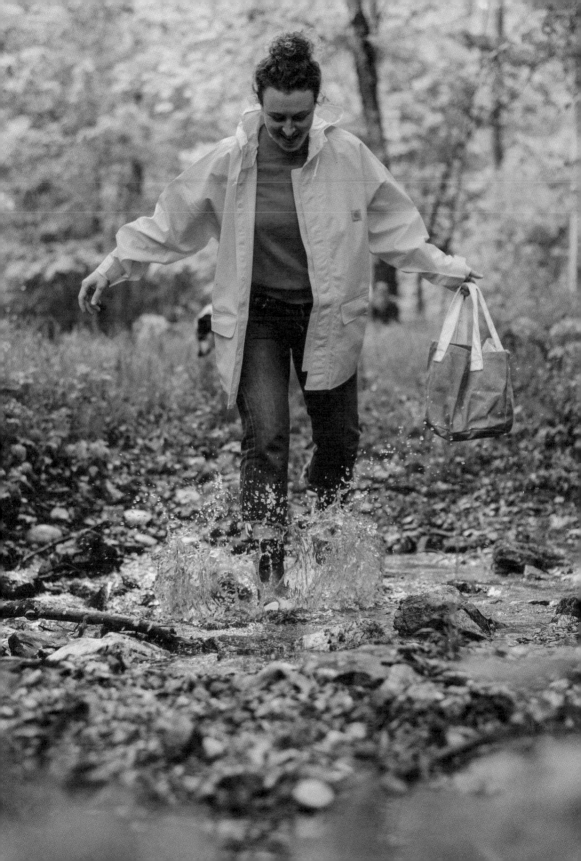

Let's Do This

Many of us move through the world unaware that the dandelions breaking through sidewalk cracks or the red clover covering highway medians are the keys to thriving in this totally bonkers world. Amazingly enough, these everyday "weeds" living in our periphery are powerhouses of resilience, generosity, and patience. Plants have evolved over 700 million years to become our best allies: they provide the oxygen we need to breathe, their ancient decomposed bodies are the fuel we burn to power our trains and heat our homes, they feed us and the animals we eat, they clothe us, and, over the years, have helped us mend everything from a broken heart to a broken bone. In their absence, we don't stand a chance. Humans have lived among plants for hundreds of thousands of years. Our deep connection and understanding of plants is recorded in our evolutionary biology, written in our family cookbooks, remembered in our home remedies, and imprinted in our DNA. Plants are not simply food, fuel, or even unwelcome garden guests: they are our healers. The beauty is that each of us can know and build an intimate relationship with plants. If this feels too woo-woo for you, consider that plants provide all of our oxygen. *All* of it. I can't think of anything less woo than the photosynthetic process. There is nothing I desire to understand more deeply than the plants that make it possible for me to breathe. I mean, not much else is happening if I quit breathing.

Look out your window, what do you see? Across the street from my Brooklyn apartment, I see a strong London plane tree growing between the slabs of the sidewalk from which loads of edible and medicinal plants sprout—including bitter dock, shepherd's purse, and wood sorrel. If I wanted to take a 15-minute walk around my city block, I could come home with a modest yet nutrient-rich meal of dandelion greens, find some plantain to soothe my summer bug bites, and gather linden blossoms for a bedtime cup of tea. Plants are everywhere, growing all around me, even in the most populated city in the United States. Presuming you are also looking out the window somewhere on planet Earth, then they are growing all around you too, from above and below.

Plants make everything possible. Here is an invitation to get to know the green world that can help us find the room and support we need to be our best most wild selves. Combined with other practices that encourage us to stretch our minds and strengthen our bodies, plants can help us change and grow. Our relationship with plants can make the world a better place in small but far-reaching ways: it can help us love the environment, love ourselves, and love one another; it can improve our health, alleviate our heavy load, and also make our meals more delicious. This book is about breaking through the wall that keeps us separated from nature and from each other. The more we know about the world around us and how to partner with the plants growing just outside our doors the more hope we may find for a happier and healthier world for all. From this place of understanding we may experience the abundant possibility of healing that plants hold.

How Does This Book Work?

This book is the gateway to the plant party just outside your door. It's about making friends with these amazing plants through herbalism—the world's oldest and most widely practiced system of healing. Through this practice, you can better understand yourself and your environment. You will learn how to center and embrace your own preferences, tendencies, and habits in the context of your health and well-being.

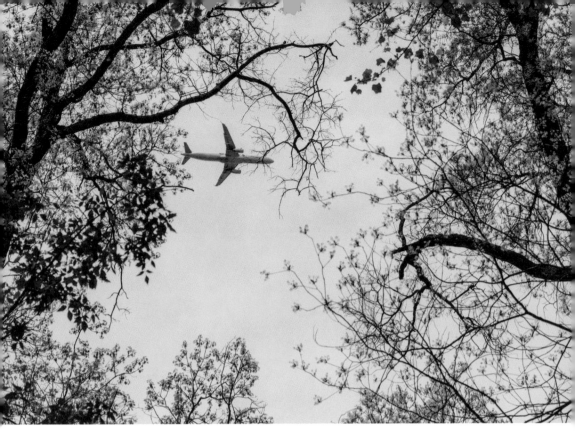

The first part of the book is the invitation to the party: It's the who, what, when, where, and why of the book. Do you have basic questions like, Who can do herbalism? What is herbalism? Where is it practiced? Can I still go to my doctor? I've got you covered.

The second part of the book is the big how, describing all the ways you can prepare to get down with plants. It is filled with practices that help you tune in and really pay attention to yourself and things to help build stronger relationships with plants: ideas to help you get outside and stay outside and the tools you need to feel at home in the outdoors. It will also teach you how to respectfully interact with plants in nature. Fields and forest are brimming with plants both large and small, some we appreciate solely for their beauty and wonder while others are wild foods. Eager to go frolicking into the wilderness armed with a basket and a wide-brimmed hat? You're not alone. Foraging can be a great way

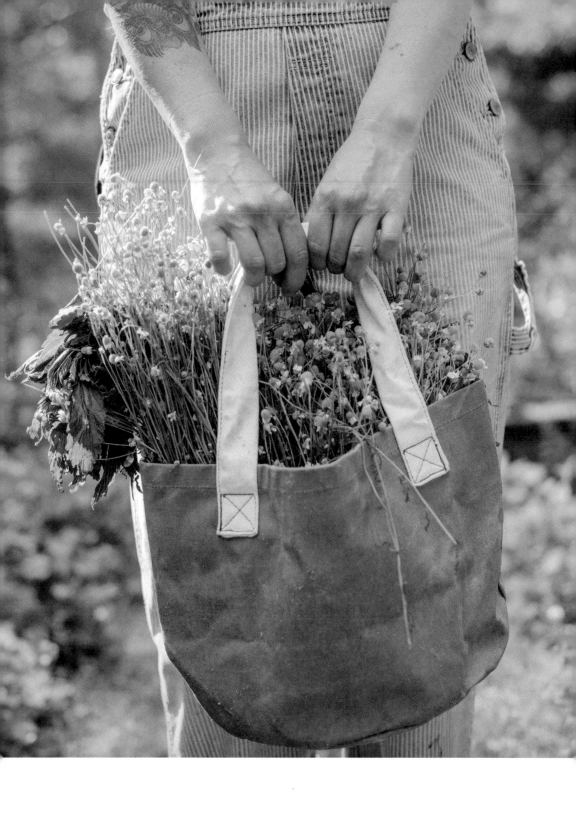

to cultivate a respectful relationship with plants and feed your supply of wild edibles at home, but it comes with great responsibility. We'll discuss what you need to consider before heading outdoors to forage and what you need to know about bringing plants into your physical home, including how to dry and store plants and prepare simple remedies from fresh or dried herbs.

Part three is your guide to everyday healing plants living just outside your door. These are the plants that come together to form a team of healing allies or your herbal arsenal. After reading through these twenty-one plant profiles you might find yourself imagining ways to politely ask your neighbors if you could please pluck the pesky dandelions from their yard so you can race home to make an oxymel from dandelion's outrageously nutritious leaves. Noticing nettle growing just inside the entrance to your local park might remind you to try a nettle infusion for those spring allergies. This book is meant to bring you back to plants and provide the knowledge, tools, and resources you need to maintain a healthy relationship with each and every one of them.

This is a book about herbalism at home; it is about welcoming the wild into your life to receive the healing of medicinal plants. It is meant to introduce you to herbalism so that you feel prepared to investigate further. If you're not ready to do it yourself you don't have to! You can always partner with someone who knows more than you. There are trained herbalists in every community, proficient in a variety of traditions, who are eager to work with you. Learning to understand when to ask for help is part of supporting our own vibrant health. There is much we are prepared to handle but in general, if your condition doesn't respond to care administered at home, including herbal remedies, within a timely manner or you feel worse, it's probably time to seek help from a professional. Any life-threatening illness or situation should be assessed, supervised, and treated by a medical professional.

Just so we're clear: I am not a medical doctor. I'm not trying to act in place of one or get you to trust me by pretending to be one. I am an herbalist. It is the law in this country and in every state that herbalists are not licensed practitioners of medicine. The information in this book is for educational purposes only. It is not a replacement for medical advice from a licensed practitioner. If you need medical care, are exploring changes to how you take care of yourself, desire medical attention, or are attempting to reach a diagnosis, consult your doctor, preferably one you can interact with in real life.

Herb Safety and Side Effects

I'm not trying to scare you, but lots of us don't know the first thing about plant identification or dosage. The good news is that herbs are generally safer than prescription medicine: they kill fewer people every year and we have a longer history of ingesting them. The United States national poison control center doesn't even have a category for people poisoned or killed by herbs because it so rarely happens. While you don't have to be terrified of the things outside your door, it's your responsibility to figure out how to identify plants with 100 percent certainty. Some plant families are safer than others—and this doesn't mean all plants within a family are the same—and with enough reading, study, and practice in the actual world you can confidently identify them. This book is not your first or last line of defense, or offense for that matter. Loads of field guides and knowledgeable people are brimming with helpful information, photographs, and illustrations. Use the old adage "look but don't touch" when assessing unknowns.

Herbalism is an art and a science; there is not a hard and fast rule for how herbs behave in unique bodies with unique genetic inclinations under a set of unique circumstances. We're all different and so are the plants that support us, and that should be a cause for celebration, not a reason to run and hide from each other, or from plants, for that matter. As with anything, start small. Simple problems generally respond to simple remedies (see sidebar page 19). Minor complaints will be easier for you to address in the beginning and are likely safe for you to self-assess with educational resources. If you get in over your head, you can always ask an herbalist.

While certain plants can have gnarly consequences when ingested or applied, none of those herbs are in this book. Those plants are toxic and are generally regarded as poisons, administered only under the care of an expert. They are different from the plants in part three, which were selected precisely for our long, safe history with them as food and medicine. You may, however, respond adversely upon ingestion or application. If you get an itchy throat or a rash or your stomach gets upset from a plant in this book, stop taking it. The discomfort will go away, if not immediately then soon thereafter.

Theoretically, any plant could contribute to a negative idiosyncratic reaction in anyone. Peanuts will kill some people, give others an itchy throat, while others

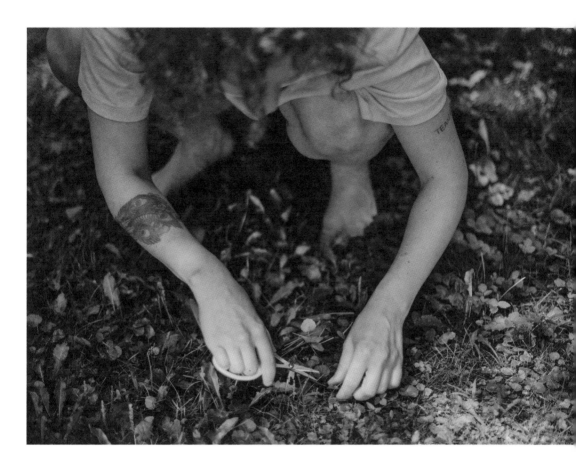

could eat a whole jar without any upset at all. When you're making choices about your health don't hand over your brain: keep it working as you read the label of a "natural" product at the grocery store or consider advice from a stranger on social media. Remember that *natural* doesn't necessarily mean *safe*, *more* doesn't mean *better*, and "it worked for them!" doesn't mean it will suit you. This isn't a plant's fault, it's not even ours, it's a natural consequence of the process of learning. Seek education from a wide variety of people and resources. Part of our responsibility in working with healing plants is to understand them and this is a lifetime's worth of work.

Healing Is a Guide Not a Goal

The point of all this herbalism chit-chat is to provide a system through which we can heal; it is not an aspirational point at which we are meant to arrive. Healing is a pathway: the more we do it, the better we get at it, the easier—and more fun!—the road becomes. Because we are not a result of healing's success or a victim of its failure, but rather a part of the process, we get to be in charge, to take responsibility for ourselves and the world we inhabit. It's tempting to think of healing as something we do outside of our day-to-day existence—as a weekend retreat or a moment of "self-care"—but healing is something we can and should be doing all the time. Healing with plants is not a vacation, as much as people would like to convince you it is; it can be demanding work that asks us to challenge assumptions about ourselves and others, systems we've inherited, boundaries we maintain or forget to hold up, and categories we rely upon to make the world a neat little box of identities and circumstances. Herbalism requires that we hold space for others and ourselves, assert our boundaries where necessary, ask for help when we need it, and find strength in connection. As a guide, the practice of herbalism can help us make decisions for ourselves with more ease and confidence. When we relieve ourselves of the pressure to "achieve health" we may find we open ourselves to many more opportunities to approach it. As a journey, healing can be a bountiful exploration of partnership with ourselves, each other, herbs, and the earth.

At the start it's important to move slowly. While a rush to the finish doesn't necessarily mean disaster, it can mean an incomplete picture. The plants in this book are safe for curious beginners to work with over time. Partner with a single plant for a month: observe it in the wild, sit next to it, touch it, taste it fresh and dried, read widely about it, but most of all pay close attention to how the plant makes you feel. Plants offer a foil to the modern impulse to skip over, skim, and speed through. What's it like to imagine change at the pace of a rose plant: season after season, year after year, rooted through sun, rain, and snow? Roses are amazing for releasing heat in our bodies and offering protection so we may open our hearts to ourselves and one another. The work of this book is to feed your curiosity about plants so you feel comfortable enough to invite them into your life every day, which will lay the foundation for a relationship with healing plants that blossoms over the course of a lifetime. Once you embark on this journey you will never stop learning, so get used to being green.

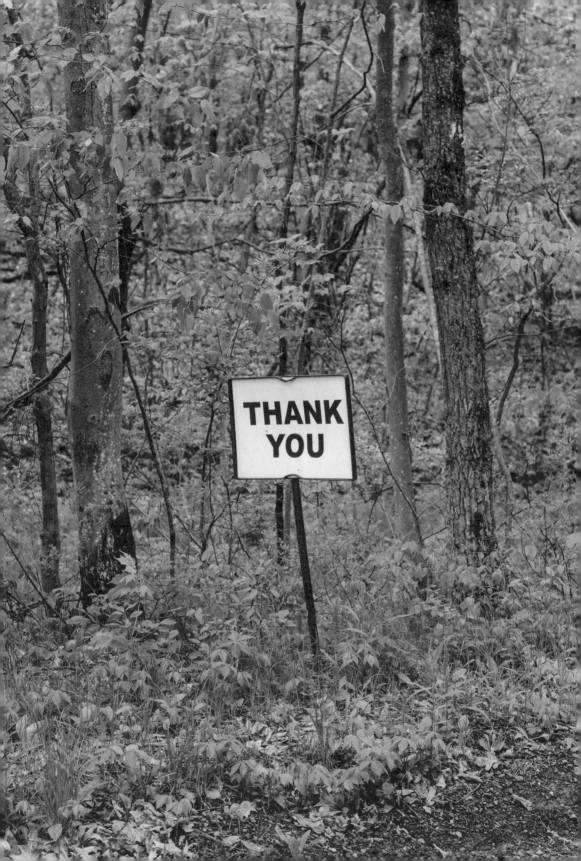

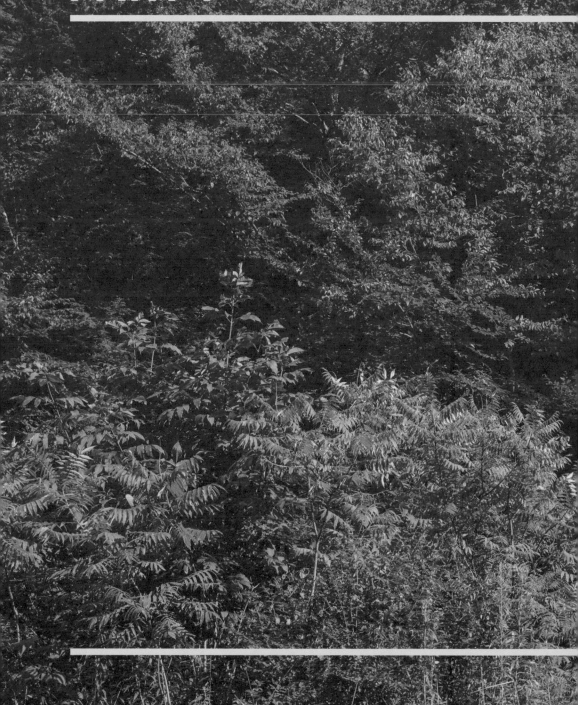

PART 1

CRASH COURSE IN HERBALISM

Next to my desk, I keep a worn printout of the front cover of a book published in the late 1800s. In bold, italicized, wanted-poster font stereotypical of the time period, it proclaims THE COMPLETE HERBALIST OR, THE PEOPLE THEIR OWN PHYSICIANS BY THE USE OF NATURE'S REMEDIES. Over 100 years later, this rallying cry still feels relevant. It's a dramatic but incredibly powerful declaration of the idea that good health, for all people, is an essential right. And with enough attention to, understanding of, and partnership with the natural world, we might achieve this for ourselves, each other, and the planet. I don't mean to suggest that we abandon the miraculous achievements of modern life, just that we don't forget about how we got here in the first place. Especially when so much of modern life makes us feel like we're not enough (social media, for one), this old book cover reminds me that the road to wellness isn't made by chasing trends. No, it's based on roughly 300,000 years of survival. It asserts that we have the ability to care for ourselves through our relationship with plants and this relationship is for *everyone*. This is at the center of our oldest system of healing: herbalism.

1

Medicine
for the People

Herbalism is medicine for the people, a system of care shaped by our needs and fulfilled by the land. We've recorded our relationship with medicinal plants since at least 5,000 BC and have an oral tradition that extends to the beginning of our time on Earth. All over the world, people continue to rely on this system. If there was any hope for the survival of the human species, the answer would have to exist somewhere in nature. And so it does: in yarrow for an open wound, clove for soothing a toothache, hawthorn for protecting and strengthening our hearts. The legacy of herbalism is present even when we try to disguise its origin as in our ginger ale and chewing gum. Plants were there at the beginning, they'll be there at the end, and it's in everyone's best interest to figure out how to invite them into all the places in between.

If we go back far enough in time, before the 45,000-square-foot grocery stores of today, we find that medicine is not so different from food. A thousand years ago things that pushed us in the direction of health didn't live on a different shelf from the things we ate every day. We don't even have to go back that far in this country to find a time when everyone did a little bit of everything and communities took care of each other, seeking the advice of "experts" only when they had exhausted all their knowledge and resources. I also want to acknowledge that many individuals and communities still do this, either by choice or by necessity. Unfortunately, in the United States, we live in a society that privileges certain lives over others and this is reflected in the institutions that govern our bodies, our accessibility to healthcare, and even in some people who are tasked at providing that care.

Our ancestors used antimicrobial herbs and spices like rosemary or cinnamon to keep meat from spoiling and ate blackberries or drank fennel tea to ease stomach upset. We all encounter acute and chronic conditions that can be alleviated with the proper plants. But we hardly need the excuse of illness or dis-ease in order to consume or apply them. We need to eat to live. And also, we eat because it provides us with the energy our bodies need to perform all the parts of being human, from building hormones to riding bikes. We eat food because it excites our senses and brings people together; it is both a profoundly nourishing and joyful act. If we trace all the food we eat back to its original source, we will end up at a plant. At one point in time and for a long time there wasn't a huge difference between what we ate, how we took care of ourselves, and the natural world from which our food and our healing remedies came. If we can leave those big grocery stores for a minute, we can see that this world is still out there. It is alive and well in the practice of herbalism.

What Is Herbalism?

Herbalism is a system of healing that relies on a foundation of good health supported by plants and food. It is a way to maintain and build robust health by making sense of our body, mind, and spirit in the context of the natural world. It's a certain way of seeing all of ourselves and each other as connected and influenced by everything around us. Put another way, each human is a living organism seeking balance. Before we go any further, let's get rid of the idea of balance as a state of stasis. Think of a gymnast on a balance beam: they are constantly moving. Even when they appear to be standing still they are flexing, readjusting, and responding mentally and physically to maintain balance. We want our own organisms to be in balance and it'd be nice if they could live in harmony with most other things, each other for example. Obviously, there's more getting in the way of that than our immediate health, but the idea of seeking balance within and on the confines of every person's epidermis doesn't have to be pretentious and lofty, or even complicated. It could be quite simple. So simple in fact, that many of us feel compelled to just paste herbalism on top of our current system of healthcare. But herbalism is much more than swapping herbs for the modern medicine we're accustomed to. Herbalism is the sum total knowledge of an entire history of our species plus the decision to trust plants and ourselves, over and over and over again. We are a part of this long history of desiring to be well, recognizing that we had what we needed to do that, honoring our curiosity, and by some stroke of luck or determination being rewarded for it.

Herbalism means that we are capable of knowing ourselves and receiving the healing capacity of nature. We don't have to be fearful of what grows in the woods, vacant lots, or our backyards. When I get worried that herbalism will ask me to adopt some kind of extreme belief system, I remember that it is simply a method of keeping myself healthy by consuming and applying plants— something our ancestors did for hundreds of thousands of years. We have made a home with these amazing plants. A home that many of us can't figure out how to honor, and yet it is still a home. In this home we too get to be part of the process of health that includes a practice of respectfully navigating the modern world. That process is called herbalism. By definition it means that we are never alone. We don't have to navigate our experiences of disease in solitude, we are always in partnership with the plants and herbs that offer healing.

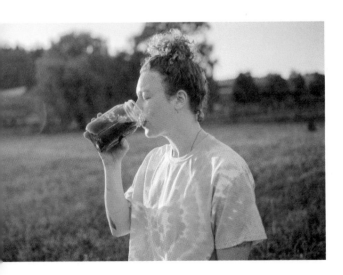

WHAT IS THE HERB IN HERBALISM?

The definition of *herb* depends on who you ask. Ask a horticulturalist and they'll tell you that herb is short for "herbaceous plant," meaning soft and green, not woody. A chef might respond that herbs are plants that season and flavor a dish; they can be used sparingly or abundantly. For herbalists, an herb refers to any plant that restores health and vitality to all aspects of the human body.

Herbalists specialize in whole plants—rather than isolated chemical constituents of plants—that support and activate the healing capacity of the body. Cedars, peppermints, and dandelions are entire systems. They have cells that build stems, leaves, flowers, roots, and seeds; cells that help them perform photosynthesis; cells that make it possible to defend themselves against predators, snow storms, and the intensity of the summer sun. Their many cells come together to taste bitter, sweet, pungent, salty, soapy, or any combination of flavors. Some cells of plants, like the hops in beer, unite to produce a relaxing, even sedating effect within our bodies while others, like the spices in chai, invigorate, envelope, and warm us. An herb is a system of many, many parts, each part dependent upon the other, all crucial to the survival of the plant itself and the good work it can do in our bodies.

WE CAN (AND SHOULD) HAVE IT ALL

The origins of healthcare, including things like allopathic medicine, midwifery, and massage therapy, share a common ancestor: herbalism. As do nurses, midwives, doctors, and pharmacists (herbalists) and modern prescription, over-the-counter, and recreational drugs (plants). Medicinal plants were among the first pharmaceuticals. In fact, the first pure, natural therapy to hit the market was an extract of morphine crystals from the latex of the opium poppy. The concentrate, named for the Greek god Morpheus for its sleep-inducing properties, is morphine.

Today, herbalism is part of an umbrella of what the World Health Organization (WHO) calls "complementary medicine," sometimes interchangeable with "traditional medicine." These two terms refer to the accumulation of all the years of knowledge and experience, beliefs and rituals that contribute to the practice of maintaining and improving the health of a population and the treatment of disease. Broadly speaking, herbalism is well-suited to promote healing through prevention by upholding the healing capacity of nature and the self-healing capacity of the body and honoring the relationship between body, mind, and spirit, and the ancestral relationship between humans and plants.

Allopathic/modern/Western medicine (whatever you want to call it) is skilled at heroic interventions. Herbalism can't be a life-saving surgery or a course of antibiotics, and that's ok. I am thankful that when my eighteen-month-old nephew's lung collapsed he had access to modern medicine with doctors and nurses who knew how to intubate him, how to administer the paralytic and the sedatives, and how to manage his withdrawal. I am thankful for the people who work in environments like a pediatric ICU who can brush up against tragedy and loss and miracles, and still commit to doing their jobs every day. Herbalism can be a way to think about and attend to an entire person as they work to uphold their health, navigate an illness, or recover at home. Herbalism can help us to remember that we are human beings who may need surgery or antibiotics and who might also benefit from flower essences to help ease the trauma of having surgery or a nourishing infusion of lymph-supporting plants after a course of antibiotics. To be clear: we need allopathic medicine and herbalism. They can be a dynamic duo instead of arch nemeses.

This is the beauty of complementary medicines—they enhance and emphasize the best of all practices, by definition. We can find support in so many ways and places, if we just open ourselves up to them. There is room for it all: allopathic medicine, homeopathy, acupuncture, counseling, psychiatry, spirituality, and the many facets of herbalism.

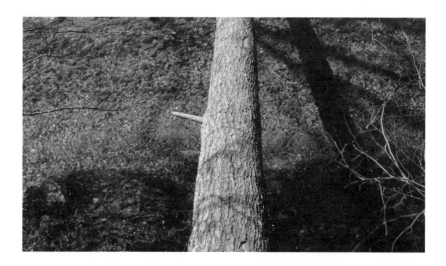

All the Herbalisms

Herbalism is practiced all over the world, every day by people like you. When choosing which system to work with, remember that many of these systems are traditions: transmissions of customs, rituals, herbal formulations, knowledge, and beliefs (plus more!) from generation to generation. Notice when you find yourself drawn to a tradition that is not your own. And ask yourself: Am I being respectful? Just because these concepts might be new to you doesn't mean these practices are, so approach with curiosity and reverence. Remember that some people may prefer not to share their tradition with outsiders and that's ok. The intersection of colonialism, racism, and white supremacy in this country are good reasons for that. Groups that have been marginalized, indigenous peoples and communities of color in particular, have experienced the delegitimization and stealing of their healing systems, been imprisoned or killed because of their traditional knowledge, and, in the case of the native populations in the United States, continue to deal with the appropriation of their ceremonies and practices plus the exploitation and decimation of their sacred plants and land. Herbalism does not exist in isolation from all the ways individuals and systems presently and historically oppress people. While you may already know this, it doesn't hurt to repeat that practicing herbalism doesn't absolve us of the social responsibility to decolonize our minds, bodies, and inherited systems of care. In fact, if we're not careful it can just be another way to appropriate and oppress communities that have been marginalized.

Perhaps the most well-known practices are Traditional Chinese Medicine and Ayurveda. The second and third largest systems of medicine, respectively, behind Western medicine. Practitioners undergo extensive training and are part of two of the oldest systems of medicine in the world. There is traditional Western herbalism, which includes folk medicine and historical uses of Western herbs. Among indigenous people of the United States are numerous systems across different Native American traditions. Many practitioners all over the world include current scientific study and research related to the use of medicinal plants. These are examples of a handful of traditions and if we were to carefully look at all populations of people all over the world in cities, communities within cities, and the ways that humans form families within those communities we would perhaps uncover as many ways to practice herbalism as there are people. When you look at all the forms of herbalism together they tend to share

ISN'T HERBALISM THE SAME AS HOMEOPATHY?

I get asked this question all the time. Usually 15 minutes into explaining the basics of herbalism, the person jumps in with "wait wait wait, so herbalism and homeopathy are *different*?" Indeed! Homeopathy is a complementary medicine founded by Samuel Hahnemann toward the end of the eighteenth century. Like herbalism, it takes a holistic approach to healing and favors the gentlest course of action first. Unlike herbalism, its founding and guiding principle is "like cures like," meaning that after a comprehensive interview with the patient the practitioner administers the homeopathic remedy that is most similar to the disease that the patient expresses. The remedy is taken in small doses to help the organism (the totality of the person in body, mind, and spirit) return to a state of health. While it's true that an herbal approach to healing may sometimes lead us to treat like with like, herbalism is neither founded on a rule of similar nor is it restricted to the use of "simples," or medicines made from single plants.

a common thread: humans have the ability to heal themselves, plants are a great way to try to do that, and it makes the most sense to respect everyone and everything through that process.

SO HOW DO I DO HERBALISM AT HOME?

When I think about answering this question, a quote from tennis player Arthur Ashe comes to mind: "Start where you are. Use what you have. Do what you can." You'll likely be surprised by how much you already know about herbalism. I'm willing to bet that you have plants in your kitchen windows, drawers, refrigerator, and cupboards. Whether you think of them this way or not, they are medicine. Their nourishment helps keep your body strong against infection and disease, they help ease minor complaints that come as part of being a human in a world full of germs and stress, and they add pizzazz to what otherwise would be a mug or stockpot full of hot water. Every time you put onions and garlic in a pot with chicken bones, root vegetables, and black peppercorns, every time you make a cup of mint tea to sip after dinner, every time you rub Tiger Balm on an achy neck, you are practicing herbalism. We may not think of these everyday, even mundane rituals as medicine, but these practices keep us fed, comfortable, and satiated with small moments of joy or rest.

Herbalism at home means attempting to adjust the big picture of our health through small meaningful acts. It is well-suited to treating minor complaints: headaches, bumps and bruises, the bitterness of a breakup, the painful loss of a loved one (ok, this falls more in the major category but is still plant appropriate), coughs and sneezes, stomach upset, and the flu. The more medicinal plants we have in our lives the more we become like them: scrappy, resourceful, flexible, and resilient. In a word: badass. I don't know about you but I want more of what-ever makes common edible plants resistant to toxic chemicals like Roundup. In spite of it all they keep on g(r)o(w)ing.

In lieu of rushing to an expert every time we get off track, herbalism is something that we can do all the time: for ourselves and with each other. We don't have to wait to get to the office of an expert, or for expensive supplies to arrive in the mail to start taking care of ourselves. With herbalism, we can start immediately, however that might look and wherever that may be. And let me assure you it will look different to each person reading this book. So long as you aren't harming other people, yourself, or the environment, there is no wrong way to do herbal-ism. There might be a *better* way, but that will come with time. Combined with adequate and restful sleep, plenty of water, exercise, time spent with people we love, and getting outside, herbal remedies can substantially contribute to our good health. We don't have to do a lot of extra work to make herbalism a part of our lives, we can simply begin by noticing where it shows up and try to be more mindful when we see that it's there. Anything we do beyond that is a big time added bonus.

WHAT HERBS (AND HERBALISTS) DO

Here are a few situations in which you might "take" medicine:

1. You have a once-in-a-while symptom.

2. You have a chronic condition.

    a. a terminal illness

    b. something that's a perennial pain in the ass, maybe even literally

3. There's an emergency.

In any of these instances, but particularly in 1 and 2b, we're used to applying the medicine to the symptom or the condition, not so much the person. In general, when we get a headache, we don't think too hard about what *kind* of headache it is, we just reach for the pill bottle. The people with the hangover, tension, or caffeine-withdrawal headache all get the same pill. There's nothing wrong with taking the pill, but the pill can only do one thing, which is to get rid of the feeling of the headache. It can't help you think about how it got there in the first place or how to keep it from happening again. Herbs don't work the same way as pills or liquids in bottles. Despite what you may have heard there's not a headache plant or a depression plant or even a cold and flu plant. Sure, certain plants are especially helpful in those circumstances, but the *person* with the headache, depression, or cold and flu is who we should really be thinking about. To many practitioners, herbalism is both a science and an art. "Treat the person, not the disease" is a popular refrain among herbalists.

There are many people, diseases, and plants. Herbalists expect that different people with different diseases will need different plants. You should too. Across herbal traditions, practitioners use systems to identify and name patterns. How we learn to apply plants to people is through a system of energetics.

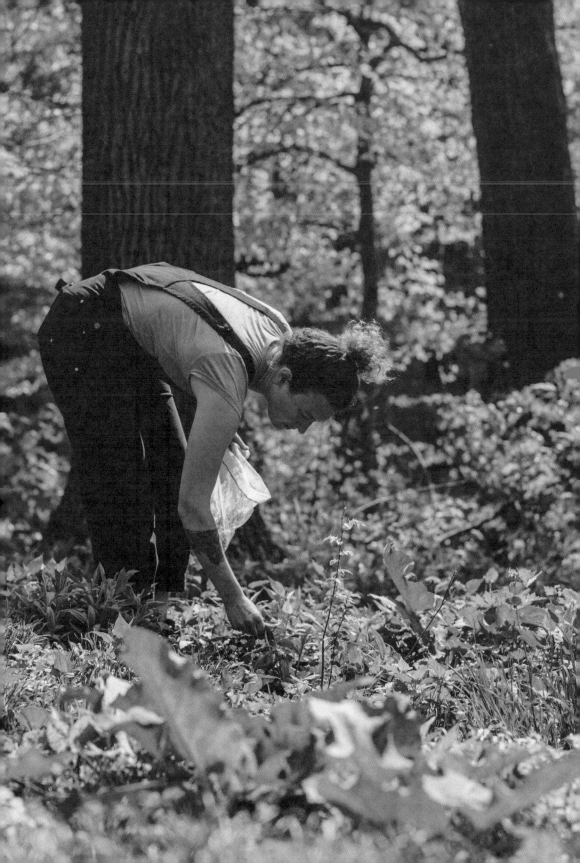

2

Energetics

Energetics are patterns. We can begin to understand energetics by simply looking for patterns in ourselves. Our ability to identify and process patterns is a unique feature of the human brain. We do this all the time, though most of the time we're not even aware we're doing it. Pattern processing makes it possible for us to read social cues, identify and remember food sources, and create and understand geographic maps. We can harness this ability to help us understand our bodies, the illnesses and discomforts that afflict them, and the plants that offer healing.

In Western herbalism we use six qualities to help classify people, diseases, and plants. Each quality corresponds to different sensations in our bodies: temperature on a spectrum of cold to hot, moisture on a spectrum of damp to dry, and structure on a spectrum of tense to lax. These qualities compose the inner and outer climate or landscape of our bodies and minds. Though they may sound like opposites, the qualities aren't in opposition to each other, but rather, rest on different ends of the same spectrum or sides of the same coin. Think of these qualities as dimensions, instead of static identities that relate to one another, whose very definition relies upon the other even existing. Even though it's helpful to have these qualities we should expect that people, plants, and diseases are apt to defy them. All of us, plants included, are skilled at challenging expectations and imposed definitions. So, anticipate that people and plants might present two qualities on different ends of the spectrum.

Your Constitution

The word "constitution" is applied when we talk about patterns in humans. These are fundamental parts of you that influence, control, and regulate what makes you *you*: the patterns that come together to form your personality, the structure of your body, and how it all feels inside your skin and in the world. There are lots of things about our bodies we can't change, a lot we inherited from the people who birthed or raised us, but there is much we can change too. Just because we were born with it doesn't mean we can't try our best to make improvements and correct imbalances. All of this contributes to forming our constitution. When we look at these things over time—days, weeks, months, or years—we see that some things come up over and over again. Identifiable patterns of physical or emotional balance or imbalance, tendencies, preferences, temperament, how our skin and hair feels and grows, and personality are some of the things that inform your constitution. Prevailing trends in your physical body or that characterize your emotions can tell you a lot about the qualities that make up your unique constitution. Your constitution is more than the symptoms listed on the back of a cough syrup or a pill bottle, or even listed in a quiz you find on the internet and in this book. You are a system of complex energies that come together to form a whole person with a unique mind and body.

Making a practice of getting to know your constitution means opening up the possibility of deeper self-awareness and acceptance. A deep understanding of your complexity and individuality has the added benefit of challenging the presumption that there are "normal" ways of being in the world, or worse "right" ways. It is my hope, and maybe yours, that practices that enlighten us about the variation of what it means to be human might bring us closer together: to ourselves and to one another. We can expect that working toward a more peaceful and just world will require a lot of change individually and collectively. The most logical place to begin, in my opinion, is by understanding how change might work within each of our own bodies and minds. This process of healing, which is more than just the solving of illness, is entirely dependent on the patterns our bodies and minds have inherited and cultivated over a lifetime.

CONSTITUTION QUIZLETS

As a way to familiarize yourself with the energetics of your constitution, try these questions on for size. These quizzes can be helpful as you begin to gather and synthesize information about your constitution. Use them to broaden your understanding of energetics and constitution. *Do not* use them as a definitive tool to explain once and for all who you are. Quizzes are fun and helpful, but they can't quite get at the nuance and specificity of each person's unique energetic framework.

Every person is composed of a mix of qualities; for example, some parts of you may be more cold or more hot even if overall your constitution is cool. If you are interested in gaining a deeper understanding of your constitution, then please work with a practitioner who is impartial and informed when it comes to assessing health: insecurities, self-doubt, and overconfidences can get in the way of really knowing ourselves. To quote Sir William Osler, "A physician who treats himself has a fool for a patient." This goes for treating ourselves at home too. Again, if your condition doesn't improve within a week, seek help. Even herbalists go to herbalists, doctors go to doctors, dentists go to dentists, and therapists go to therapists.

For the following quizzes, you have two simple choices: A or B. If you believe strongly that you're somewhere in the middle, then you probably are. For simplicity's sake I chose to illuminate what the ends of the spectrum look like so that you can not only understand yourself better, but the degrees of energetic qualities as well. Like I said before, qualities exist on a spectrum and they go something like this:

TEMPERATURE: Hot—Warm—Neutral—Cool—Cold

FLUID: Very Dry—Dry—Neutral—Damp—Very Damp

STRUCTURE: Relaxed—Neutral—Tense

Try to pick the extreme that you feel closest to. If you get stuck while reading the questions it can be helpful to think of how you were as a child and the patterns that you've sustained for most of your life, especially in regard to physical traits. If it feels too overwhelming to go back to childhood to answer questions that pertain to behavioral patterns, then just answer in regard to the last few years. Again, this is not the be-all and end-all of your constitution exploration. Resist the urge to rely on this quiz to help you figure out who you really are. And instead, use it as a general guide to what long-standing patterns you might have.

HOT AND COLD

1. GOING TO BED, I TEND TO
a. throw the covers off and open the window; I am a tiny furnace.
b. wear socks and reach for my hot water bottle.

2. WHEN I'M UPSET, I USUALLY
a. get red and excited. I may raise my voice or even stomp around.
b. retreat, make myself small, and keep relatively quiet.

3. IN LARGE GROUPS
a. I feel like I can be opinionated. I don't mind and even like attention. I am comfortable chatting with strangers.
b. I am most comfortable with people I know, in a side room talking quietly.

4. WHEN HAVING A MEAL
a. I often get seconds.
b. I usually leave food on my plate.

5. WHEN I THINK ABOUT "TAKING THE DAY OFF," I
a. panic: "Relax?! You mean *do nothing*?!"
b. can't wait: Great! I have just the pajamas for this sort of thing.

6. WHEN I HAVE AN HOUR TO MYSELF I AM MORE LIKELY TO
a. exercise.
b. do something quiet indoors.

7. WHEN I GO HOT TUBBING
a. I am desperately searching for the spigot of fresh, cool spring water.
b. I am first in, last out.

Tally your choices: an abundance of As points toward more heat while an abundance of Bs is in the direction of cooling qualities.

DRY AND DAMP

1. MY WATER BOTTLE
a. is with me all the time, I drink from it and refill it often.
b. is usually left behind at home. Coffee has water in it, right?

2. MY NAILS
a. grow slowly and break often.
b. are naturally long and strong.

3. A STEAM ROOM
a. is my idea of heaven.
b. is my idea of hell.

4. IN THE MIDDLE OF AUGUST IN A HOT CITY
a. I'm not even breaking a sweat.
b. I'm like a soggy sponge and have a change of clothes with me at all times.

5. I AM MORE LIKELY TO COMPLAIN ABOUT
a. the scaly patches on my elbows.
b. my acne.

6. I TEND TO HAVE
a. an itchy scalp and dandruff.
b. oily hair.

7. WHEN I MOVE
a. I can feel and hear my bones crunching or cracking.
b. I do so without too much restriction in my muscles or noise from my bones.

Tally your choices: an abundance of As points toward more dry qualities while an abundance of Bs is in the direction of damp qualities.

LAX AND TENSE

1. IN GENERAL
  a. I alternate between work and rest effortlessly.

  b. I can take a while to transition out of work mode.

2. AT BEDTIME
  a. I start my bed routine without much resistance and am out when my head hits the pillow.

  b. I have a hard time getting to sleep. What was that thing I wanted to google?

3. TO HELP MY BODY RELAX
  a. I book a deep tissue massage.

  b. I like to stretch.

4. I AM MORE LIKELY TO COMPLAIN ABOUT
  a. diarrhea.

  b. constipation.

5. MY VEINS
  a. are prominent.

  b. . . . what veins?

6. MY GLANDS
  a. . . . glands? Where are they? I don't really think about them.

  b. are swollen and even kind of hard.

7. MY MUSCLES ARE
  a. relaxed and twitchy.

  b. tight and dense.

Tally your choices: an abundance of As points toward more lax qualities while an abundance of Bs is in the direction of tense qualities.

Use your answers to help you identify where you might fall in regard to the following table. The table can further assist in your identification of patterns within certain parts of your body. It also lists remedial plants, including those found in this book. These plants are best suited to the type of constitutional qualities you exhibit in your body and mind. The quiz and the table can help point you toward the plants that might best make up your team of wild plants, what I like to call an herbal arsenal.

CONSTITUTIONAL CHART

QUALITIES	HOT	TENSE	DRY
QUICK REFERENCE	This person or tissue state is overly excited or stimulated.	This person or tissue state is constricted or tight.	This person or tissue state is depleted in oil and water or both.
PATTERNS	Irritated, red, swollen or inflamed tissues that are hot to the touch Excited/excitable Stimulation/stimulated Nervousness Difficulty sleeping Fever "Sharp" pain Sensitivity to pollution, allergens, other things in the environment	Restricted range of movement Shaking, spasm Psychological nervousness Physical or psychological tightening and tension Some characteristics tend to fluctuate between extremes like fever with chills or appear to come and go suddenly like diarrhea	Cracking joints Constipation, bloating Thin hair that breaks easily Weak or shriveled skin, tissue, or muscle Scant urination Scaly, itchy skin
REMEDIES	Cooling plants that slow down or sedate tissues or functions. **Rose, hawthorn, lemon balm, elder, peppermint, chickweed**	Relaxing herbs, generally aromatic, that soothe and reduce resistance within the body and mind. **Chamomile, catnip, peppermint, linden, lemon balm**	Moistening plants that soften and tone the system. **Violet, cinnamon, linden, red clover, plantain, catnip, chickweed**

COLD	RELAXED	DAMP
This person or tissue state is slow to respond to stimulation and prone to underactivity.	This person or tissue has lost its ability to contract and tone.	The fluids in this person or tissue state are backed-up and accumulating.
Pale complexion Feels cold when others aren't Cold toes and fingers Bloating or constipation Prone to infection and low-grade fevers Generally tired Foggy, slow thinking "Dull, achy" pain Depressed function	Bleeding gums Excess perspiration Cool, clammy skin Lacking firmness and tone Spongy or swollen tissue Excessive flow of fluid can lead to overall drying effects in the body	Impaired energy Improper elimination function Poor digestion Weight gain Dull facial expressions Slow wound healing Feeling "hung over" from eating or drinking or just because that's how you tend to feel
Plants that encourage and increase function through stimulation or increasing circulation. **Ginger, garlic, thyme, white pine, rosemary, cinnamon**	Astringent herbs that tighten and tone tissue. **Sumac, rosemary, plantain, white pine, rose, hawthorn, elder**	Nourishing plants that improve flow throughout the body, especially in regard to digestion. **Dandelion, red clover, nettle, cinnamon, plantain**

Patterns in Plants

Herbs and plants are as alive as we are. They begin, grow, reproduce, and die. They have environments they like and times of year they prefer. They are dynamic beings full of vigor and influence, all of which we can feel. Plants have energetic qualities: hot, cold, dry, damp, lax, tense that assert actions on and in our bodies. They also have another element of taste: sweet, sour, salty, bitter, spicy, savory, pungent, acrid. A plant's taste can tell us a lot about its energetic quality. For example the sweet taste of rose indicates that it's cooling. The pungent quality of thyme tells us it's probably good at moving things in our bodies. The salty, earthy taste of nettle points toward its high vitamin and mineral content. The combination of a plant's qualities and tastes contribute to what herbalists refer to as "herbal actions" or how we experience plants in our bodies: feelable, identifiable, describeable habits of a plant in a human body. We can tell through our senses if a plant is astringent like an unripe banana, demulcent like the slippery infusion made from marshmallow water, or a digestive aid like the bitter dandelion leaf. Like qualities, plant actions aren't in opposition to one another and actions that sit on different ends of one spectrum (relaxing or stimulating, for example) might very well reside in the same plant.

Understanding Plant Actions: Matching People and Plants

Employing energetics and plant actions provides a common language from which to work together: people with plants and people with people. Each plant tends to have general benefits, but the particulars of how those benefits might be felt depends on the person feeling them. We all feel and experience things differently, this includes the imprint of plants on our senses. What feels hot to me might be warm to you or potentially even cool. So, the combination of a person's constitution and the quality of a plant's actions are not only how we feel but also how we describe the feeling. This means that while we can expect the astringent action of sumac to tighten and tone tissues in our bodies, how much and in which location will not always be the same person-to-person or even within the same person every time.

It's worth trying to understand what "action" an herb encourages in our body and how it achieves it but resist the urge to assign outcomes to plants (i.e., echinacea is the cold and flu herb or St. John's wort is the depression plant). When we do this, we remain open to experiencing the actions of a plant in our bodies by turning our attention to what a plant does best and how that feels to us: finding our own language to describe our relationship to the astringent, bitter, stimulating, demulcent, or diaphoretic actions of a plant. This is counterintuitive to the way we currently think about "getting better," which is almost always asked in the form of How can I stop _____ from happening? When we work with herbs, instead we ask, Which plants might best support me right now by moving me in the direction of balance? The answer to this question is found in the plant's actions, which we can determine through our senses. These are examples of the habitual expression of the plant, and they can tell us a lot about what it will do in our body and even how it might do it.

Cultivating an intimate understanding of plants and how they work in your body can help you facilitate what your body is already skilled at: nourishing and supporting the systems that keep us alive, fighting illness, and working toward a state of harmonious health. In understanding plant actions, we liberate ourselves from being overly reliant on the expertise of other people and from alleviating symptoms without ever getting to the root of what ails us. Our bodies are equipped to run a productive fever to fight a virus, induce a runny nose to keep out pathogens, and rush blood to a wound to fight infection. Learning the actions of plants can help us pay attention to and trust that our bodies are skilled at healing.

HERBAL ACTIONS

The following definitions are intended to be a quick reference to the myriad ways plants work within and on our bodies. This list is not exhaustive (it accounts only for the plants in this book), and these terms do not apply exclusively to plants.

ALTERATIVE: herbs that restore proper eliminatory function, thus increasing health and vitality. You might hear these called blood builders or purifiers.

ANALGESIC: herbs that reduce pain.

ANODYNE: herbs that relieve pain.

ANTICATARRHAL: herbs that prevent inflammation of the mucus membranes and dissolve and remove mucus from the body.

ANTIFUNGAL: plants that prevent fungal growth.

ANTI-INFLAMMATORY: herbs that reduce and relieve inflammation inside or on your body.

ANTIMICROBIAL: herbs that destroy a wide spectrum of pathogenic organisms including bacteria, fungus, and virus.

ANTIOXIDANT: a substance that inhibits oxidation and eliminates free radicals.

ANTIRHEUMATIC: herbs that protect against and resolve symptoms that result from disease affecting the joints, muscles, or connective tissues.

ANTISEPTIC: herbs that prevent the growth of infectious, disease-causing organisms.

ANTISPASMODIC: herbs that prevent and ease spasms or cramping in the body.

ANTIVIRAL: plants that protect against or reduce the lifespan of viruses (not all viruses or antivirals behave in the same way).

AROMATIC: plants high in volatile oils with pleasing odors that calm through the digestive and/or nervous system.

ASTRINGENT: herbs that reduce secretions and discharges by contracting tissue.

BITTER: herbs that tone and stimulate the digestive system.

CARDIOTONIC: herbs that tone and strengthen the heart.

CARMINATIVE: herbs that help expel gas from the stomach and intestines (most of our common kitchen herbs and spices).

CHOLAGOGUE: plants that promote the secretion of bile from the gall bladder.

CIRCULATORY STIMULANT: herbs that improve the circulatory system to help blood flow through tissues.

DECONGESTANT: plants that help alleviate congestion.

DEMULCENT: herbs that are high in mucilage and soothe irritated or inflamed tissues.

DIAPHORETIC: herbs that encourage perspiration thereby improving elimination of toxins through the skin.

DIURETIC: plants that work on your kidneys to increase the amount of salt and water that comes out in the flow of urine.

EMMENAGOGUE: herbs that regulate or promote menstrual flow.

EMOLLIENT: herbs that soothe and soften to protect the skin.

EXHILARANT: herbs that uplift the spirit.

EXPECTORANT: herbs that help the body expel mucus from the respiratory system.

HEPATIC: herbs that support and promote liver function.

LAXATIVE: herbs that stimulate bowel function.

LYMPHAGOGUE: herbs that promote and stimulate lymph flow.

NERVINE: herbs that act on our nervous system to calm and soothe anxiety and stress.

NUTRITIVE: herbs that support by nourishing usually by filling nutritional gaps in our diet.

RELAXANT: herbs that reduce tension and promote relaxation.

RUBEFACIENT: herbs that when applied topically stimulate circulation locally.

SEDATIVE: plants that calm the nervous system strongly, often inducing sleepiness.

STIMULANT: herbs that stimulate the nervous system.

STOMACHIC: plants that strengthen the stomach and support digestion.

TONIC: generally nourishing, gentle herbs that strengthen and tone a specific tissue or organ. Tonics are generally qualified with specific types (astringent, liver, etc.).

TROPHO-RESTORATIVE: herbs that strengthen and nourish a specific organ or tissue so much that the accomplished improvement or restored function lasts even after the use of the herb is discontinued.

VASODILATOR: herbs that dilate the blood vessels.

VULNERARY: herbs applied topically that help heal wounds.

WHAT'S THE DOCTRINE OF SIGNATURES?

The doctrine of signatures says that herbs that look like certain parts of the body or conditions treat ailments of those organs, systems, or conditions. For example, the shape of pine branches and needles is a signature for our respiratory system. While Dioscorides (the ancient Greek physician) was one of the first people to write about it, that doesn't mean it wasn't being thought about and practiced all over the world at the same time, which is true for a lot of the history of herbalism. Plant signatures appear in Traditional Chinese Medicine as a concept and in certain Native American traditions. It was popularized in Western folk medicine during the Middle Ages. While the doctrine of signatures can be true for some plants, is a handy mnemonic device for remembering the actions of plants, and is an interesting piece of history, I believe that it is an incomplete and not necessarily clear picture of a plant. Also, it's hardly the only way of understanding a plant in any of the aforementioned modalities. But to dismiss herbalism due to the doctrine of signatures is just as unfair, and frankly stupid, as dismissing the practice of Western medicine because three physicians bled George Washington basically to death. At the same time, simply saying that the leaves of lungwort look like lungs and are therefore good for the respiratory system doesn't accurately represent a whole picture of a plant and also limits our understanding of a plant as an entire system. To herbalists, there's another way of looking at an illness: a set of circumstances acting on and within the human body.

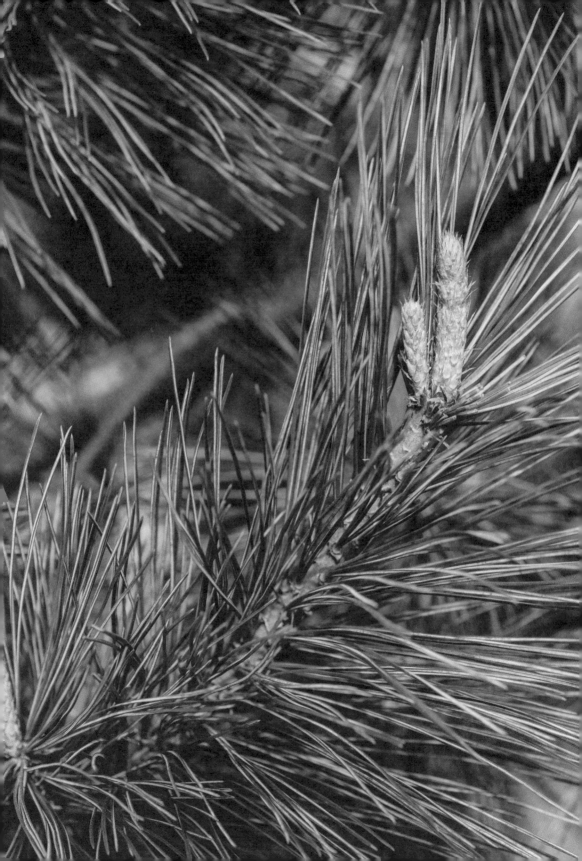

PART 2

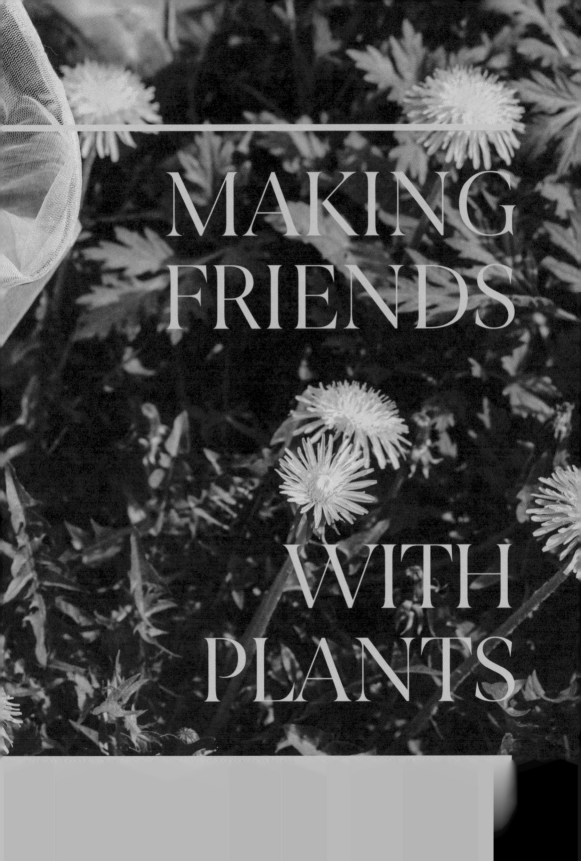

MAKING FRIENDS

WITH

PLANTS

The best place to make friends with plants is on their own turf. Maybe you're hesitant about getting out there. It's a wide, wild world and after hundreds of thousands of years of working so hard to move our homes indoors we've gotten pretty comfortable on the couch, so to speak. Rest assured, you are built for the outdoors.

This section is about getting on that plant level, getting used to their speed, their turf, and them in general. We'll discuss ideas for slowing down and prioritizing joy—two essential ingredients to not only reducing stress and anxiety to bolster our health but also to learning about plants. You will understand how to work with plants better if you are having fun. Be light! No discussion about being outside with plants is complete without a pep talk on stewardship! So that's all in here too: establishing best practices so we are sure to have them around for generations to come. And what about bringing them into our world? That's in this section too: everything from a better cup of tea to a medicinal salve. I've got you covered inside and out.

3

It's a Plant World, We're Just Living in It

Somewhere between 450 and 475 million years ago the first organisms to live on land full time moved out of the ocean. After washing ashore, their evolution was likely slow and arduous, with setbacks and casualties along the way, but they did it. Can we focus on the immensity of this moment for a second? Plants growing on land is one of the most important evolutionary breakthroughs in the history of the universe as we know it. These anatomically simple plants were the first organisms to effectively immigrate, and their survival depended upon the success of the relationships they would form. So that's what Earth's first plants did: they made friends.

Earth's first land plants didn't have deep roots: they had neither an extensive root network, nor a long line of ancestors from which to draw adaptive mechanisms and favorable traits for survival. These first plants populated areas not far from water, often right up against it, as it would have been impossible to survive beyond a moderately wet environment. Plants made allies with fungi, letting them live on and in their roots in exchange for food and water.

This relationship would later be coined *mycorrhiza* meaning "fungus root" by Polish scientist Franciszek Kamieński. This symbiotic relationship is hundreds of millions of years old and still going strong today. Had it not been for fungus living in the soil, land plants would have been without an adequate food and water supply to eventually acquire the adaptive traits they would need to grow and spread. Vascular systems and the ability to produce seed to populate everywhere from arid plains and mountainsides to lush tropical forests and fertile valleys to crevices of walls and ruins of forgotten buildings were all dependent on this crucial partnership. It is what enabled plants to develop stronger roots, grow taller to compete for sunlight, develop seeds and cones, and form relationships with pollinators like bees, moths, bats, birds, and butterflies.

Today, the plant world still includes non-vascular plants—likely among the first land plants—like mosses, liverworts, and hornworts, clubmosses, spikemosses, and quillworts; vascular plants like ferns; gymnosperms or "naked-seeded" plants including spruce, ginkgo, yew, and cycad; and angiosperms or "vessel-seeded" plants like roses, oaks, palm trees, cacti, orchids, corn, and sunflowers. Altogether about 300,000 known species of plants exist on Earth. Thanks to that moment in time when plants and fungi started working together.

They don't need us, but we need them. As autotrophs, plants create their own food. Through the process of photosynthesis they harness the energy of the sun, using it to convert water and carbon dioxide into sugar for food that drives all of their necessary cell function so they can contend with disease, fend off predators, compete with other plants, and reproduce. In turn, plants are the beginning of every food chain and web on the planet. Everything we eat starts with a plant. The same process, feeding oneself, that costs us outrageous amounts of physical energy, money, and time plants do for free. It is in our best interest to understand them. Without us they'll go on living, but without them we may cease to exist. It behooves us to protect and serve them. This part of the book is about getting to know plants better: understanding their environment, learning how to respect them in their habitats, and respectfully engaging with them to heal ourselves and the environment we share.

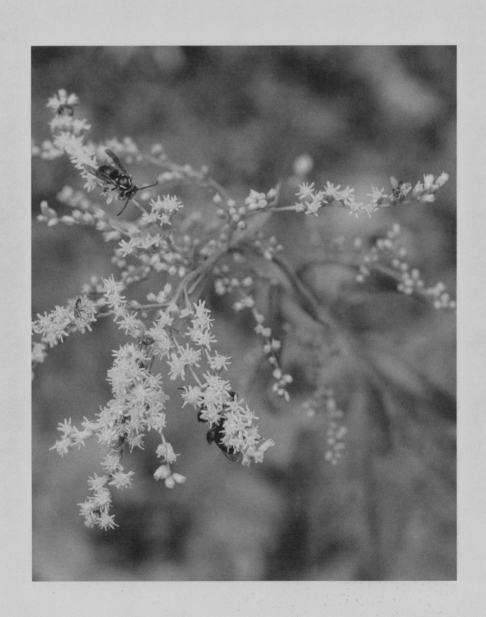

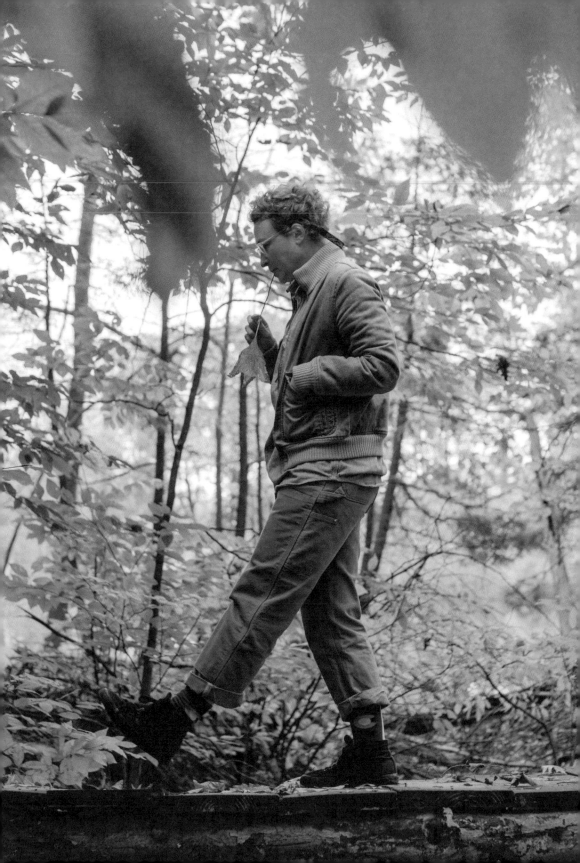

Go Outside, as Often as You Can for as Long as You Can

Lots of scientific articles begin with the sentence, "There is growing evidence to suggest that exposure to natural environments can be associated with . . ." insert benefit of being outside. Growing evidence? Really? As if the longevity and advancements of an entire species and all the things that live outdoors that gave us life aren't evidence enough. Why in the world are we looking to experts to confirm what we already know in our bones: being outside is good for us.

The outside world is full of things we need to live: water, sunshine, plants, and fresh air. The good news is that all your green friends (your allies!) are outside. In forests, bordering the rivers and diving canyons nestled among the towering mountains of California grow giant sequoias, older than anyone on Earth by a long shot, that defy gravity every day by pumping water 250 feet into the air. In the patch of grass between your apartment building and the sidewalk is the dandelion whose relative came over on the Mayflower. In a dewy part of your city park grow native succulents. In the arid plains of the West grow sacred white sage plants. At the New York Botanical Garden in the Bronx, north of Manhattan Island, a dwindling population of native hemlock trees survives in a small piece of untouched American continental forest that has never seen a logging truck. And pressing up against the chain-link fence of your neighbor's yard is the sweet rose, whose scent will uplift and open our hearts asking us to connect more deeply with ourselves and to make the same attempt with the wide world. Endeavor to return the eagerness of their generosity, be brave enough to embody the fearlessness of their vulnerability, get to know them. Extend them the trust and gratitude they've demonstrated to the rest of the world. Get out there, it's all waiting for you.

Ok, I'm Outside . . . Now What?

Congratulations! You did it.

The following ideas are meant to inspire you to engage with the plants in part three, and even the ones beyond the pages of this book. The more time we spend outside the more confidence we gain in the company of plants and in identifying them. Here are recommendations on where to go, what to do, and things that might be useful once you're out the door.

PLAY

Forgot how? Watch some kids for a second. Cultivate boundless joy, however you can or want. Sit. Laugh. Walk. Laugh. Run. Laugh. Roll. Laugh. Gather your friends and spend a day in the park or on the beach. Only don't just sit there: explore. Look up into the trees and down at the earth, pause to wonder and gently touch. Funnel sand and soil through your fingertips. Spend a long time watching the clouds, tides, bees, caterpillars, spiders, ants, birds, and worms. The habits of natural phenomena, insects, and animals can teach us much about the natural rhythms of our environment. Familiarizing ourselves with the patterns of nature means that we have another clue to the habit of a plant: the seasons in which they begin to grow, bloom, and die. This helps us understand what times of year they may be most beneficial. The gentle bitterness of young dandelion leaves in spring, for example, can ease us back into eating raw foods after a winter digesting root vegetables and heavier cuts of meat. Being joyful outside with plants means we can receive knowledge about them with ease, allowing for a deeper understanding that unfolds over time.

INVEST IN FIELD GUIDES

Many people have gone to the effort to compile written descriptions and visual depictions of flora into handy, transportable books. They range in variety: Some are heavy on botanical language, others are colloquial. There are vintage guides and modern guides, some with illustrations, others with photographs. Being alone in nature with a field guide might be the slowest way of teaching yourself to identify plants but learning how to use them is a worthwhile skill in itself. Field guides are essential tools to helping us identify plants with 100 percent accuracy,

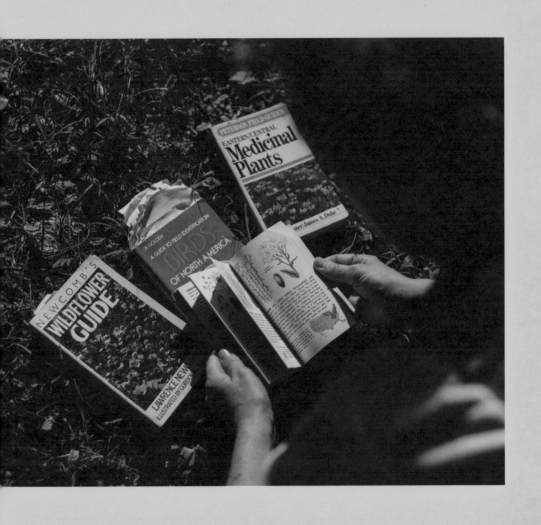

which is your responsibility and yours alone. Not to mention they are filled with fascinating information including scientific facts and folk tidbits. A field guide will provide you with detailed descriptions of all of the plants in this book. Before you head out in the world, familiarize yourself with the plants that grow in your area. Find a few field guides that communicate and illustrate poisonous plants in a way that makes sense to you. Use the knowledge to inform your own method of recalling the plants as they become more and more familiar to you—the physical markers that differentiate myriad species of rose, for example, or how to tell the difference between stinging nettle, wood nettle, and clearweed.

LEARN FROM PEOPLE WHO DO THE THING

There is always someone who knows more than me and is excited to share what they know. Probably the case for you too. I love these people. My favorites are birders, naturalists, mycologists, other herbalists, botanists, farmers, historians, and elders. These people are skilled at watching the world go by: they practice observation as often as possible wherever they are. For those of us who are used to talking all the time, getting outside is a good opportunity to shut up, watch, and listen. Attuning ourselves to the migratory patterns of monarch butterflies or Canada geese can tell us a lot about the plants in bloom at a particular time of year. Understanding the mushrooms in an environment can tell us more about the climate there and the plants that may be found nearby. Talking to the farmer can teach us a lot about weather patterns and what foods to expect at the market at what time of year. Enriching our understanding of the pacing of the seasons through any of these means can only help deepen our grasp of the ebbs and flows contained within the organs and boundaries of our own organism: the human body.

GROW PLANTS IN YOUR HOME

Getting everything we need from shrink-wrapped Styrofoam, inside a cardboard box, or out of a shiny plastic bag sounds like a lousy way to live. It means a lot of junk is going into our bodies and the landfills, probably even the ocean. Why are we looking for health in yellow-five-hued syrup? Or paying $60 for vitamins? That same amount of money could buy at least ten plants that could live in your home or garden. Many medicinal plants, such as thyme, parsley, oregano, and mints like lemon balm, grow fine indoors in a sunny window. They provide the ingredients to make a tasty tea or broth that is rich in the vitamins and minerals your body needs to grow strong, as well as remedies for a headache or a sore throat. Also, caring for plants can help us tune in to how we care for ourselves. When I'm feeling reluctant about watering my plants it generally corresponds to a reluctance to take care of myself. Picking away dead leaves and paying attention to watering preferences reminds us that it's worth taking time to care for something, especially yourself.

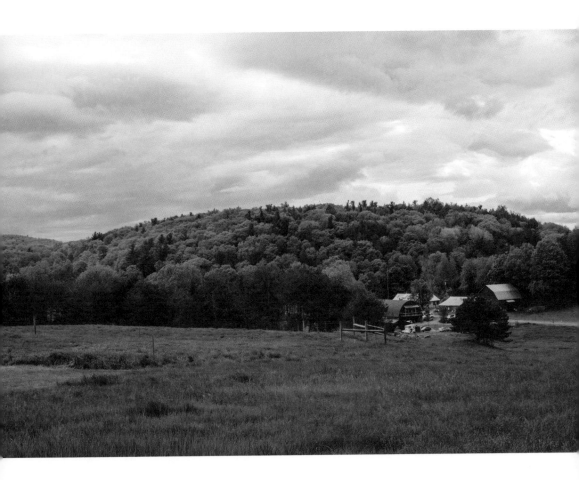

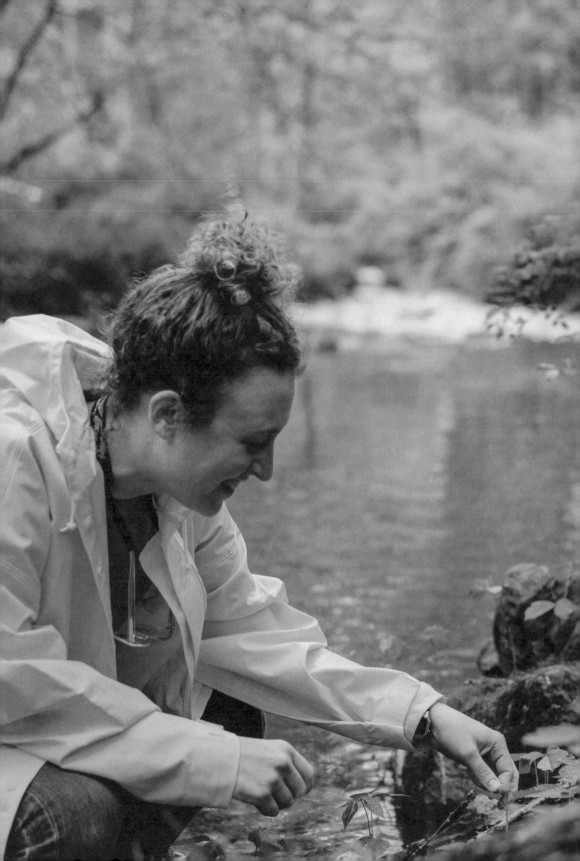

4

The World of Wild-Crafting

Where to begin? There is so much going on outside: ecologically, socially, politically. And it all gets thrown together in a basket, canvas tote, or a brown paper bag when it comes time to have a conversation about wild-crafting. Wild-crafting—or foraging—means harvesting non-cultivated plants from the, you guessed it, wild. They might come from forests, fields, vacant lots, or public land.

I'm going to assume that you aren't reading this book because you're interested in commercial wild-crafting. What we're discussing here is how to supplement some of the medicinal plants you purchase or grow in your home with wild edibles. These include common weeds like ground ivy, dandelion, and plantain that re-establish themselves easily as well as non-native plants, like garlic mustard, which have negative allelopathic effects on surrounding plants.

Why Wild-Craft?

Why in the world would you want to forage in the first place? For one thing, we don't get a lot of wild food in our lives anymore. Though we've spent most of our evolutionary history gathering our food, we are presently out of touch with a practice that kept us in rhythm with the natural world. So, with the following suggestions in mind, here we go!

STEWARDSHIP IS NUMBER ONE

This land is your land, this land is my land. Our relationship with plants is foremost one of stewardship and we should make that our priority when thinking about wild-crafting. Our primary concern should be taking care of what's around us to prevent overharvesting. Observe what you intend to wild-craft for at least a year (a what?! Yes, a year) so that you have a good idea of who else uses the plant on which you've placed your heart and mind. Take a mental or better yet, an actual photo of the area you're inspecting, ensure that it looks the same when you leave as when you got there. Be discreet and mindful of limiting damage to an ecosystem; as a general rule never harvest more than 10 percent of a healthy population. Remember that animals, birds, insects, fungi, other plants, and people rely on many of the same things that you do. The blueberries aren't just for you, they're also for the robins. And the roses are for bees and butterflies too. You might show up one year to what is ordinarily a bountiful elderberry harvest and find that only a handful of berries hang on. There's just not enough for you to take a share this time. That's ok! More and more small farmers are cultivating medicinal plants. Their work needs our support. Also remember that wild-crafting could mean not just picking plants to take home, but also helping save seeds of endangered and at-risk plants and relocating those plants whose habitat faces destruction: plants that grow in the path of residential or commercial development, for example. There are lots of ways to be a friend to plants.

YOU ARE ON STOLEN LAND

Through war, trickery, loop-holed treaties, and just plain old stealing, white people systematically took this land away from Native Americans. YIKES! If you aren't indigenous to this country, this is not your ancestral land. Consider what it means to be a good guest in someone's home: be on your best behavior, don't take up too much space, keep things as they are, ensure that things look better when you leave than when you got there, be grateful, be helpful, give thanks. We have a responsibility to care for our shared home. We can use how we interact with native and non-native flora and fauna as a way to work through the devastating consequences and lasting effects of colonialism. Those of us with colonizer heritage can make better choices than our ancestors did and we can do all of that as we explore the outdoors. Questions to consider might include: How can I support the preservation of indigenous plants for the populations that need them most? Which native flora could I plant in my garden or community garden? Which plants should I avoid wild-crafting? How can I ensure I'm not purchasing from disreputable sources?

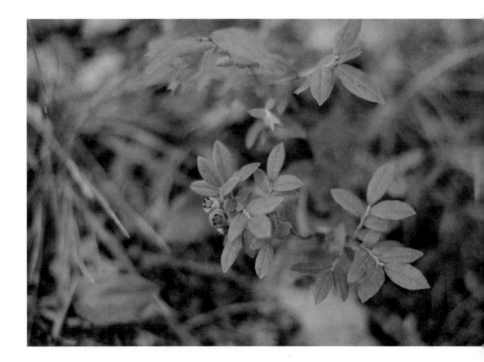

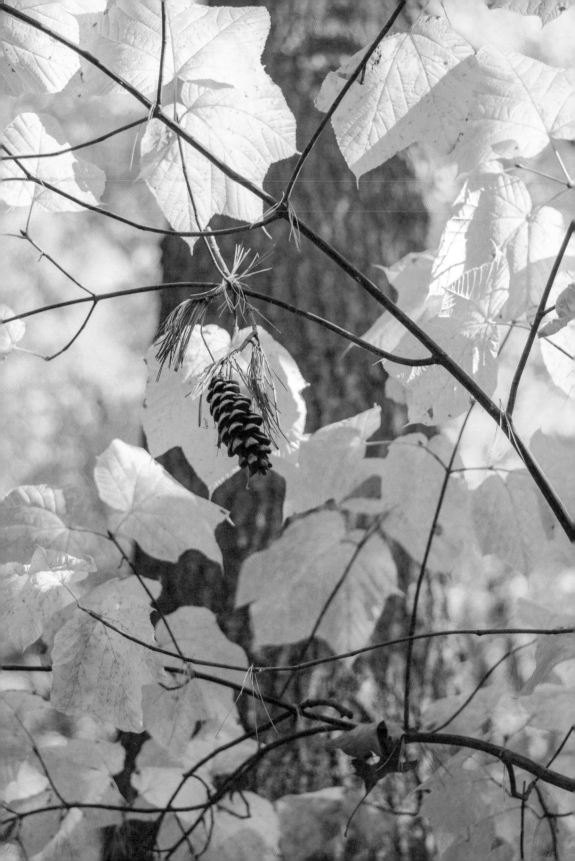

ASK PERMISSION

This might go without saying, but the amount of true public land in the United States is small and, sadly, getting smaller, so ask permission of landowners where appropriate. What I'm *really* interested in though is asking the plant for consent. This might mean you will sometimes hear a "no." And if you're always getting yes, perhaps you're not listening close enough. It's possible that you go out in the world and come home empty handed this time because no one said yes. I know I've spent a large part of this book reassuring you that these plants are for you, so to suggest that we ask permission may seem like I'm contradicting myself, but plants don't *belong* to us. Just like humans, they are their own beings. If talking to a plant sounds absurdly silly to you then maybe think of it this way: you are meeting this being for the first time, on their turf, don't assume anything and take some time to get to know them. If asking permission brings up too much discomfort, then you can just sit—they'll be happy to have your company!

KNOW YOUR ENDANGERED AND AT-RISK PLANTS

In order to familiarize yourself with at-risk and endangered species spend some time on the United Plant Savers website. Use your field guide to see if any of the plants on their endangered and at-risk lists live in your area. Decide that these are the plants you will absolutely never harvest not even "just this once." Be a model of stewardship to anyone else who joins you outside. What's more: don't buy any of these plants if someone is selling medicine made from wild-crafted versions of them. In fact, be thorough in investigating anyone selling wild-crafted plants or medicines. Find a farmer and sign up for their Community-Supported Agriculture (CSA) or join a community garden instead. Use field guides to identify which plants and which parts of them you are meant to harvest, which habitats they prefer, and the times of year they grow.

Field guides can also help you identify equivalent plants you might look for in place of overharvested ones. If you understand how different plants propagate, you may decide to leave the seeds and roots of certain plants untouched.

SIT WITH IT

When in doubt just take a knee or a booty or whatever. Stay still and watch, breathe, observe. This might sound totally out there but you don't even have to ingest a plant in order to reap its benefits. Cozy up to the base of an oak tree, kneel in a field of yarrow (check for ticks if you're in the Northeast), sit cross-legged in the red clover. Look up, look down. Be quiet, and if you're familiar with meditating, do that. Check out who else might be enjoying the sights and sounds. Consider that a plant may ask nothing of you, except perhaps to honor it. It's ok if you're not sure exactly what that means, but don't rush to push past the discomfort. Stay awhile with that feeling and see where it takes you.

BE SAFE

If you're looking for something to fear in place of poison ivy try pesticides and herbicides. Avoid harvesting in heavily manicured locations, under power lines, or near railroads. Be sure you're not collecting downhill from where waste is deposited or near open sewage. For urban dwellers: be mindful of the pollution that our plants endure. While I don't want to discourage you from picking *any* plants in a city, I think it's good practice to avoid places close to traffic and exposed to chemicals especially. Remember that Superfund sites exist in cities and much of our soil contains contaminants like lead. Some of my favorite and most reliable places to forage are the interior of our beautiful public parks. If you're unsure of where to go, look for a naturalist in your area who leads walks.

If you live in a place where ticks live, check for them! Look on and underneath your clothes for these tiny insects, sometimes smaller than a poppy seed. It's better to get to them before they latch. When you remove a tick from your body that hasn't attached make sure you pay attention to where you put it once it's off your body. It would be silly to sling it into the surrounding area and then walk back into it as you leave. Who on earth would do that? Not me, never.

HELPFUL TOOLS FOR THE OUTDOORS

- Field guides with both written and illustrated or photographic descriptions
- Mesh or recycled plastic bags for transporting plants home
- A tote bag or basket for collecting plants
- Scissors for more tender parts of plants
- Clippers for branches or woodier plants
- A small knife
- Camera or phone
- Tick and bug repellent
- Notebook and writing utensil
- Water
- Tall socks, closed-toed shoes
- A loupe to inspect things more closely (flowers close up are wild!)
- A handkerchief

My go-to plants to forage from this book include:

- Chickweed
- Dandelion
- Plantain
- Red clover
- Catnip
- Sumac
- Linden

Bringing Plants Home

So what to do with these fresh little green things? Whether they come from the market, your community garden, or the wild, processing and storing fresh plants properly means that less of them end up in the compost pile before their time has come. Remember that the more you bring home the longer you'll spend cleaning, drying, cutting, and storing or cleaning and immediately preparing medicines. Our eyes are often bigger than what our bodies or refrigerators are prepared to hold, so it's better to feel like "Dang it, I didn't get enough!" than "Dang it! Another bundle of lemon balm in the compost pile." Learning this lesson is heartbreaking. So, having been there, take my word for it: less is truly more.

If it's not too humid where you live you can hang your fresh herbs in small bundles out of direct sunlight or spread them out on a clean screen held aloft by two supports or suspended over drying racks in tiers. Remember that different parts of different plants are the most medicinal and to make your life easier you may want to do some work before you dry them, like plucking chamomile flowers from their stalks, for example. Plants can and do get moldy in the process of drying or in storage so be sure plants and jars are completely dry before storing. It could take a couple of weeks before the plants are dry enough to snap at the thickest parts of their stems. If you live in a humid place, like much of the Eastern United States and Midwest in the summer months, consider investing in a dehydrator. If your oven runs at 180°F or less then you can safely dry your plants in a single layer on a baking sheet, if you want to have your oven on in August that is.

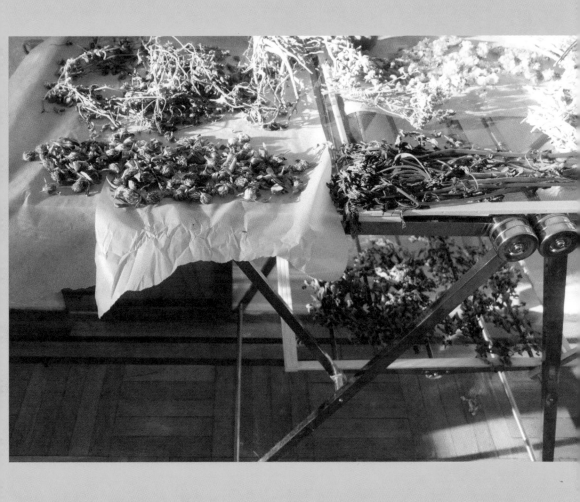

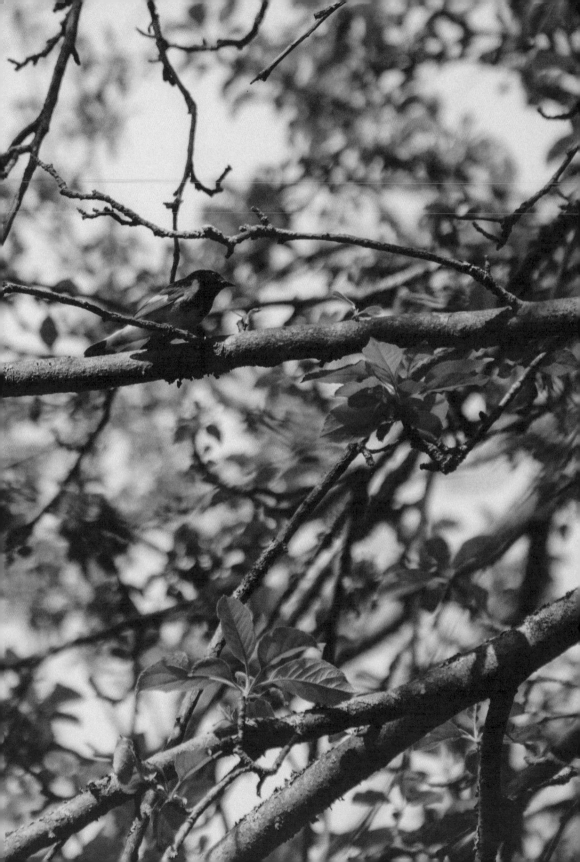

5

Making Medicines at Home

Making simple medicinal preparations from familiar plants doesn't have to be a big to-do. You probably already have everything you need to get started and if you don't it can be acquired swiftly and affordably. Self-reliance is the name of the game when it comes to preventative healing. Not to be confused with "doing it on your own," reliance on oneself is primarily about trust: honoring an awareness and understanding of yourself. Read all of the instructions *before* you start making things. This way you can be sure you have what you need and the time to do it. Some preparations require you get started 24 hours in advance and some require a month for part of the recipe.

It is in your best interest, as well as that of the planet, to support best practices. Whenever possible buy plants, oils, beeswax, honey, maple syrup, and other products from local farmers who grow without herbicides or pesticides (many farms forgo the official "organic" designation, but this doesn't mean they aren't technically farming organically). More and more herb farms are cropping up, many of which offer seasonal herbal CSAs—these are great ways to familiarize yourself with the seasonality of a plant and to get to know new-to-you plants. Refer to the resources section at the back of this book for some ideas of small farms and producers that offer online purchasing or offer local pick-up and delivery locally. And remember, of course, that many of us work within a predetermined budget or the confines of our geographic location. The best we can do is the best we can do.

Tincture

A tincture is a concentrated extract of a plant in a menstruum (liquid) like alcohol, apple cider vinegar, or vegetable glycerin. While I prefer infusions and decoctions for preventative and chronic situations, tinctures can be taken in lower doses over extended periods of time for chronic conditions and in higher doses for acute situations. Tinctures can be incredibly helpful in situations where you need something immediately or you don't have access to a kitchen. You can take a tincture on a plane, on the subway, in line at the grocery store, or at your desk. **Yield varies depending upon herb type and whether you use fresh or dried forms.**

Fresh or dried herb of choice

Alcohol, apple cider vinegar, or vegetable glycerin

1. **Finely chop the aerial parts of a fresh herb or use a mortar and pestle for tougher parts** like dried roots or rhizomes.

2. If using **fresh herbs fill a quart size jar about halfway up**. Don't pack them in as they'll expand as they absorb the water from the menstruum. If using **dried herbs fill the jar about one-fourth the way up.**

3. **Cover the herbs with your chosen menstruum**. The formal ratio of menstruum to fresh herbs is 2:1 (weight:volume) and the ratio of menstruum to dried herbs is 5:1.

4. **Use a chopstick or another skinny stirring device to swirl the liquid around**. Cap tightly and shake. It's important to prepare and store tinctures made with vinegar in a vessel with a lid that won't corrode; if you don't have a BPA-free plastic lid then line the top of the jar with plastic wrap.

5. **Label your tincture with the date and ingredients.** I also like to add where the herbs came from: "Sawmill Herb Farm, MA" or "Cyd's Garden," for example. This helps me stay connected and remember why I made the medicine in the first place. Leave a bit of space on the label for the date you will eventually strain and store the tincture. The layout of your label might look like this:

"Herb" in "menstruum" from "location"

Date made

Blank space for the date you strain and store the tincture

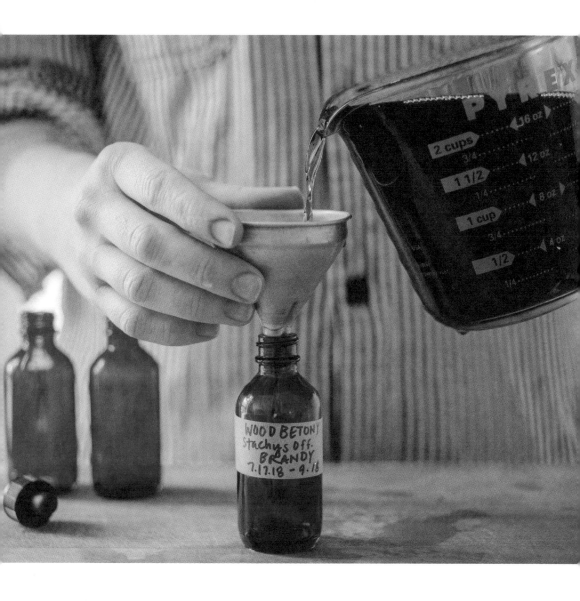

6. **Check back the next day.** Dried herbs will absorb the menstruum, so you may have to add a little bit more liquid so that the plant material is covered completely by about an inch of menstruum and swims freely. Store out of direct light in a cool spot that isn't out of sight. You want to remember to shake the tincture-in-progress every day so things don't settle and all the bits stay moving and extracting.

7. **After 4 to 6 weeks, strain, compost, and store.** Use a fine-mesh strainer (lined with cheesecloth if you want) to strain the liquid from the solids. Squeeze and press the liquid from the strained herbs and compost the plant material. Store the tincture in an amber, green, blue, or clear glass bottle (I prefer "Boston Round" bottles—see the resources section at the back of this book) in a cool, dark place.

As a reminder not all plants are meant to be ingested; some are intended for topical use only. Also, remember that not all parts of the same plant do the same thing. It's a good general rule to consult a few resources if you're unsure. Don't take just one person's word for it, including mine.

WHICH MENSTRUUM SHOULD I CHOOSE?

You have three choices: alcohol, apple cider vinegar, or vegetable glycerin. For home remedies an 80- to 100-proof alcohol—like brandy, vodka, or gin—has enough water and alcohol to extract the medicinal properties from the herb. Tinctures prepared in apple cider vinegar or vegetable glycerin are not as strong (which just means you will need to take larger doses if you're a larger person), but they are appropriate for children and folks who prefer to avoid or have sensitivity to alcohol. Traditionally, tinctures made from glycerin are known as glycerites and are well-suited to herbs like peppermint, ginger, dandelion, chamomile, and nettle. Apple cider vinegar tinctures are most appropriate for plants with high mineral content like nettle and dandelion as well as cinnamon, peppermint, and rosemary. Additionally apple cider vinegar and glycerin are considerably more affordable than alcohol.

HOW LONG DO THEY LAST?

Alcohol tinctures keep almost indefinitely. If you make a large amount don't store your tincture in a dropper bottle because the alcohol can erode the rubber over time. Instead, keep it in a glass bottle with a tight-fitting cap. Glycerin tinctures will keep for a few years and apple cider vinegar tinctures for about a year.

HOW MUCH DO I TAKE?

The plants in this book are safe to take 30 to 60 drops 3 times per day.

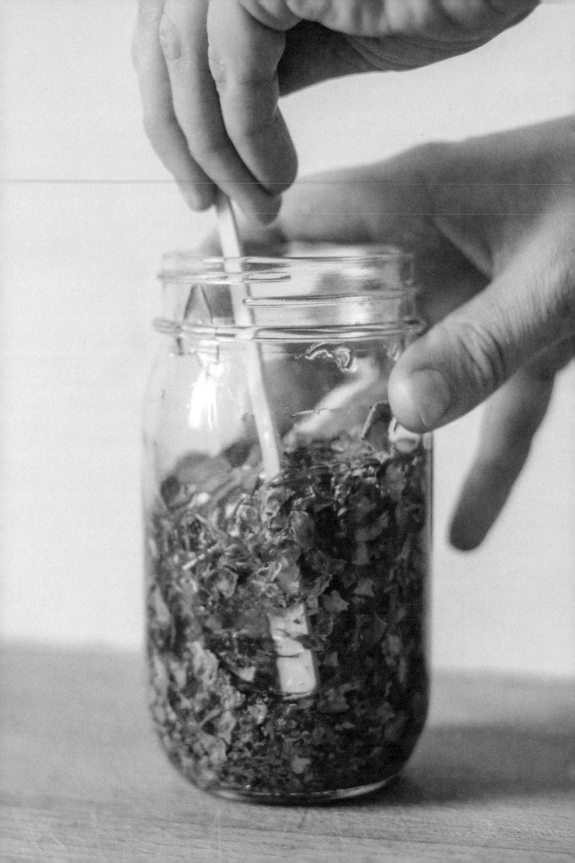

Herbal Honey

An herbal honey preserves any part of and delivers the medicinal actions of a plant in a naturally tasty, nutritious, and medicinal substance. Herbal honeys are powerful double medicines that are simple to prepare and delicious. Honey is one of our oldest naturally occurring medicines and modern research supports its broad-spectrum antimicrobial activity. When we ingest or apply herbal honeys we receive the power of the herbs infused in the honey as well as about 200 other substances that occur naturally in honey, including probiotics, vitamin C, and B vitamins. Honey is an effective remedy for inflammation on or inside the body: topically for burns or internally for sore throats and even stomach ulcers. My favorite herbal honeys for topical burns are rose petal or lavender flower honey. Thyme-infused honey, sometimes with a little powdered clove, is my go-to for sore throats. **Makes about 2 cups.**

WHY CHOOSE LOCAL, RAW WILDFLOWER HONEY?

When we choose local, raw wildflower (or pesticide-free single flower) honey we tap into our local ecosystem and economy. Go to your farmers market and talk to the beekeepers. They are knowledgeable and generally happy to discuss their work caring for honeybees, which are responsible for pollinating almost $30 billion a year in crops in the United States alone.

2 cups local, raw honey

About 1 cup fresh or dried herb of choice

1. If you're using fresh herbs—before chopping—leave them out to wilt for 8 to 24 hours and up to 3 days (depending on the time of year, humidity, and type of plant) before adding the honey.

2. **Warm the honey until it is a pourable consistency.** Set a saucepan of water over low heat until it is about 100°F, turn off the heat, and set the honey (which should be stored in a glass jar) in the warm water for 10 minutes so that it thins to a pourable consistency. The temperature of a honeybee nest is kept between 92°F and 98°F, so you can warm the honey to roughly human body temperature without damaging its integrity. If it's hot outside and hot in your apartment you likely won't have to warm it up.

3. **Roughly chop the aerial parts of a fresh herb or use a mortar and pestle for tougher parts** like dried roots or rhizomes.

4. **Add the herbs to a glass quart jar** (fresh herbs will fill two-thirds of the jar and dried herbs half of the jar).

5. **Pour the warm honey into the jar.** It should cover the herbs completely so that when you tip the jar everything swims around with enough room, like in a glitter wand. Use a chopstick or another narrow stirring device to remove any air bubbles. Add more honey if needed and be sure to cap and label the jar.

6. **Put the jar on a plate and flip it upside down and back every few days**—or a couple times a day if you're really committed—to ensure everything is getting soaked with honey. If using fresh herbs, the honey's consistency will loosen as the water is extracted.

7. **After 2 to 4 weeks your herbal honey is ready.** If you want to decant the honey to separate the herb, then warm the entire jar in warm water like you did in step 1 and use the strainer to pour off the honey from the plant solids. But don't compost yet! Pour hot water over the honeyed herb to make an instantly delicious tea or infusion. I usually just keep everything together in the original jar. If I plan to use the honey topically, I'll just strain off a bit especially for that purpose.

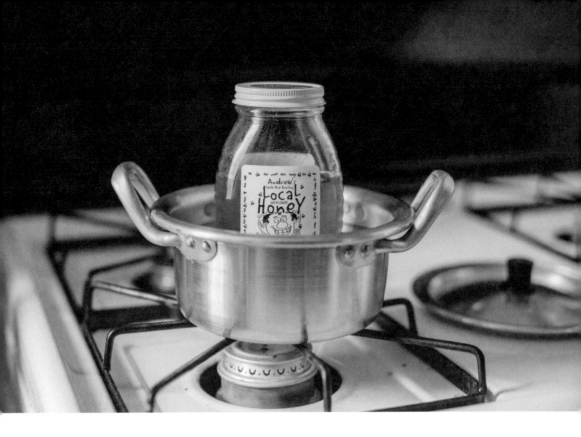

HOW LONG WILL HERBAL HONEY LAST?

Herbal honey made from fresh plants won't last as long as honey made from dried plants, which will last indefinitely. To ensure the longevity of a fresh plant herbal honey keep it in the fridge; since it's more liquidy than regular honey it will likely maintain a suitable consistency for spoonfuls at cooler temperatures. Overtime, especially if exposed to cooler temperatures, your honey might crystallize, but this doesn't mean it's gone bad. Honey can even crystallize in the hive in the late fall through the early spring. If you want to get back to that smooth spot just warm the honey back up either with the warm water method, in a double boiler, or just heat your spoon up before dipping into the jar.

Oxymel

An oxymel is a sweet and sour medicinal preparation made from herbs, honey, and apple cider vinegar. More than 2,000 years ago the father of clinical medicine, Hippocrates, proclaimed, "Let food be thy medicine," and also prescribed oxymels for respiratory disorders.

Oxymels are a combination of two preparations we've already discussed: tincture and herbal honey. Since ancient times oxymels have been popular medicines for diffusing and expelling anything that needs to get out: a cold in your chest, gas in your stomach, or headaches (for instance, like a chamomile and rosemary oxymel when I have a caffeine-withdrawal headache). Though they are shelf-stable, I keep many in my refrigerator because I like how they taste cold.

Oxymels are tasty on their own or when added to other beverages. If you find holiday family gatherings anxiety-inducing (as many people do), carrying around a 1-ounce bottle of lemon balm oxymel means you can instantly transform any favorite alcohol or soda water into a tension-taming medicinal drink. **Makes about 1½ cups.**

1 cup local, raw honey

1 cup apple cider vinegar

1 cup dried herb of choice (double for fresh)

1. If you're using fresh herbs, leave them out to wilt for 8 to 24 hours and up to 3 days (depending on the time of year, humidity, and type of plant) before you begin.

2. **Warm your honey until it is a pourable consistency.** Set a saucepan of water on the stove on low heat until it is about 100°F, turn off the heat, and set the jar of honey in the warm water for 10 minutes so that it thins. The temperature of a honeybee nest is between 92°F and 98°F, so you can warm the honey to roughly human body temperature without damaging its integrity. If it's hot outside and hot in your apartment you likely won't have to warm it up.

3. **If using fresh herbs, roughly chop the aerial parts of a fresh herb or use a mortar and pestle for tougher parts** like dried roots or rhizomes.

4. **Add the herbs to a glass pint jar** (fresh herbs will fill two-thirds of the jar and dried herbs will fill half of the jar).

5. **Add equal parts warm honey and apple cider vinegar to the jar.** Whether you want your oxymel to be sweet, tart, or perfectly balanced is up to you. Oxymels are totally customizable to your

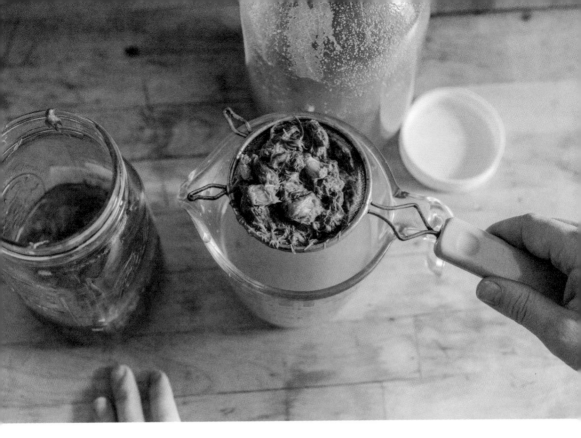

preferences or for whomever you are preparing the oxymel. More honey for sweet, more vinegar for tart. Experiment and have fun. Label and cap the jar with a plastic lid or metal lid plus wax paper or plastic wrap.

6. **Shake well and set out of direct sunlight on top of a plate to catch any drips.** Continue to shake every couple of days to ensure everything is getting equal honey-vinegar attention.

7. **After 2 to 4 weeks your oxymel is ready! Strain, compost, and store.** Use a fine-mesh strainer (lined with cheesecloth if you want) to strain the liquid from the herb solids. Squeeze and press the liquid from the strained herbs and compost what's left over. Store the oxymel in an amber, green, blue, or clear glass bottle in the refrigerator. It will last for 1 to 2 years, if you can successfully ration your intake for that long! Chances are you'll go through smaller preparations in a couple of months at which point it will be time to make more of the same or something new.

Medicinal Tea

A medicinal tea is a pumped-up cup of tea. It can be a single herb or a combination and is created for a specific purpose with healing in mind. This simple preparation soothes me after a rough day, is an excellent companion during a difficult phone call, and helps me maintain good practices around winding down from my day. A moment with a cup of tea is especially helpful in times of transition: everything from getting into bed to getting out of a relationship.

Ask yourself some questions before choosing your herb. Are you going to sleep? Trying to clear your head? Maybe you have a stuffy nose? Are you drier than usual? Was today a stressful day? Preparing a cup of tea is primarily an opportunity to check in with yourself: how does your body, mind, and spirit feel? Preparing a cup of tea provides a moment to respond positively to how we might be feeling in a small dose. **Makes 1 serving.**

1 to 3 tablespoons herb(s) of choice, roughly chopped if fresh

1 cup water

Honey or sugar (optional)

Milk of choice (optional)

1. **Fill a tea ball infuser or mug-sized strainer** with your herb or herb combination and set inside your mug.

2. **Boil the water.** Wait just a few seconds before pouring the water over the plants. In my opinion just-boiled water is too hot for many plants and diminishes the tastes.

3. **Pour the water in the mug, cover with a plate, and steep.** Allow about 4 minutes for highly aromatic herbs like chamomile and peppermint, and between 7 and 10 minutes for almost anything else.

4. **Adjust to suit your preferences, breathe in, and sip slowly.** Add sweetener and milk of any variety, if desired. Remember medicine can be a treat, not a punishment.

Infusion

An infusion is basically a strong tea over time: an extended steep of the aerial parts of a plant in water. Infusions use more plant matter than you usually would for a cup of tea, generally 1 ounce of herb to 4 cups of water. If you don't have a kitchen scale, not to worry, you can use a dry cup measure as a guide. You can make hot infusions or cold infusions, depending on what is most appropriate to the plant you're infusing. I like to prepare most of my nourishing infusions in the evening while I'm putzing around my kitchen tidying up. **Makes about 3 cups.**

1 ounce or 1 cup of dried herb (double for fresh)

About 4 cups water

Heatproof quart glass jar or teapot with a lid or a top, or a French press

Strainer or cheesecloth

Another mug or glass to serve

1. **Boil the water, if desired.** This step is optional. As a general rule I prepare hot infusions, though lots of plants can infuse in cold water, even chamomile and peppermint.

2. **Measure 1 ounce of dried herb or 2 ounces of fresh** if using leafy parts, a little bit more for flowers (they're bigger and fluffier and take up more space with their sprawling parts), and a little less if infusing fresh roots or rhizomes. Add the herbs to a heatproof glass quart jar, teapot with a lid, or a French press.

3. **Pour the water over the herbs** and cap lightly if using a jar. Don't screw the top on and never shake the jar (you will give yourself a terrible burn). Let it infuse on the counter for 30 to 40 minutes until it's cool enough to touch.

4. **Set the infusion in the refrigerator and let steep for 4 to 12 hours.**

5. **Using a mesh strainer or cheesecloth (or both), pour off the liquid from the herb.**

6. **Store your infusion in the refrigerator** as it will spoil over time, especially if it is hot indoors and you're using mineral-rich plants like nettle or red clover. The refrigerator is also a good place for infusions of roots and barks like marshmallow or cinnamon whose demulcent actions activate in cold water. If these plants are part of a recipe including plants that require a hot infusion, it's ok to begin the whole thing in hot water. As the infusion cools in the refrigerator, the mucilage in something like marshmallow root, for example, will activate in the colder water.

INFUSE OR DECOCT

As a general rule, the more delicate parts of a plant like leaves, flowers, seeds, and some fresh berries are infused, because boiling these tender things can potentially damage and render the medicinal qualities unusable. While this is not a hard and fast rule, most roots (dry or fresh) and dried berries can be decocted (see page 75).

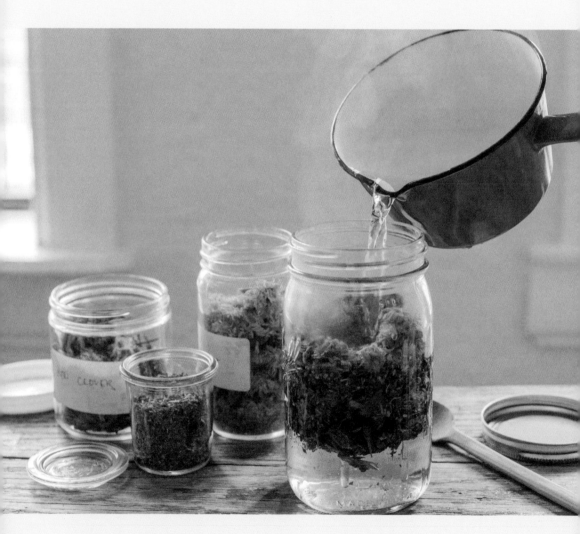

LUNAR AND SOLAR INFUSIONS

If you're interested in harnessing the energy of the moon or the sun, let them shed their light on your infusions. Prepare your infusion as usual (if you're doing a solar infusion and it's the hot summer you don't necessarily need to preheat the water). Leave the cap off the jar you prepared your herbs in, put a piece of cheesecloth with a rubber band over the top to keep the critters out and put your infusion in the light of the sun or the moon during the day or while you sleep, respectively. In about 12 hours your galactic brew will be ready!

CLASSIC INFUSION COMBINATIONS

Not sure where to get started? Here are some tried-and-true herbal combos: plants that are friendly in action and pleasing to those with which they're paired. Each combo includes at least one or two plants in this book.

- Nettle leaves + peppermint leaves + licorice root or marshmallow root (simple nourishing infusion that's not too drying)

- Catnip leaves and flowers + passionflower leaves + chamomile flowers (midday soother)

- Plantain leaves + calendula flowers + peppermint leaves + marshmallow root (herbs for gut health)

- White pine needles + thyme leaves + citrus zest (warming winter brightener)

- Sumac berries + tulsi leaves + hibiscus petals (cooling summer sipper)

- Violet leaves + nettle leaves + dandelion leaves + mint leaves (spring has sprung tonic)

- Peppermint leaf + lemon balm + lemon verbena + maybe some green tea if you're feeling wild (summer coffee substitute)

- Rose petals + linden flower + lemon balm (comfort from your close friends)

- Linden flower + elderflower + lemon balm (transition tea)

- Red clover + oat straw + mint (sweeten with honey for a nourishing infusion)

HOW LONG DO I LET MY INFUSION GO?

How long to infuse depends on what parts of what plant you're using, but the longer you steep the stronger the infusion. This is true for the strength of *all* the constituents you extract: it will be stronger in vitamins and minerals and also likely in taste. As an experiment, prepare 2 cups of chamomile tea: 1 tablespoon of dried flowers to each cup of water. Pour the boiled water over the mugs and cover with a plate to keep in the aromatics. Taste one cup of tea after 5 minutes and the other after 30 minutes. What do you notice? Possibly that the cup you steeped for 5 minutes tastes like chamomile tea: smells a little appley, is pleasantly floral without being too sweet. It would go down incredibly easy if it wasn't so hot. The one that steeped for 30 minutes, however, is likely so bitter that that's about all you can taste (this doesn't mean it's gone bad, it just means it's taken on another medicinal level).

HOW LONG DO INFUSIONS LAST?

In general, 3 to 4 cups of infusion per day is the recommended dose. If you can't finish it all in one day, store any leftovers in the refrigerator so it won't spoil and try to finish within 3 days.

WHICH PLANTS IN THIS BOOK SHOULD I INFUSE?

Catnip	Lemon balm	Red clover
Chamomile	Linden	Rose
Chickweed	Nettle	Rosemary
Elderflower	Peppermint	Sumac
Fresh ginger root	Pine needles	Thyme
Hawthorn flower	Plantain	Violet

Decoction

A decoction is a low and slow simmering water extraction of the more fibrous plants and fungi like mushrooms or parts of plants like seeds, berries, roots, and bark. So many plants make perfect decocting plants! Onions and garlic (technically leaves), reishi or shiitake mushrooms, burdock, astragalus, dandelion root, cardamom seeds, and elderberries. There are also lots of popular pot-herbs, leafy additions for your decoction, like the fibrous stalks and leaves of fresh nettle or sea vegetables like kelp. You can add these at the beginning or the end of the decoction depending on how fibrous they are. A decoction can be anything from a savory broth or a rich, chocolatey, spicy-sweet drink. My favorite thing about a decoction is you can make huge amounts at once, a great way to unite your herby friends and your people friends. If you've prepared a large pot of decoction, you can just leave the pot on the stove and invite people to help themselves with a ladle and a small mug-size strainer. You can keep the heat on low and continue to add more water or just turn the heat on if it cools.

Fresh plant matter contains more water, so it will naturally dilute the decoction as it releases its own water content. You always have the option to make your pieces smaller by using a mortar and pestle or spice grinder. I generally just throw everything in so long as it's all roughly the same smallish size. **Makes 4 cups.**

1 ounce or 1 cup roughly chopped dried herb (double for fresh herbs) or about ¼ cup (1 tablespoon dried herb per 1 cup water)

4 cups cold water

1. **Combine your herbs and water in a 2-quart saucepan.** I was taught to start any decoction in cold water. And by decoction I mean stock, which is essentially a decoction of roots, other fibrous vegetables, and some kind of animal or fish bone and flesh. This is because certain proteins are only soluble in cold water, whether they come from an animal, fish, or plant.

2. **Turn the heat to low, bring to a gentle simmer, and cover.** The key words here are low and slow. We are going for a long simmer to produce a strong decoction. There is no rush. You'll likely have to turn the heat down even lower once you put the lid on so that it doesn't bubble over. I like to simmer most decoctions for 30 minutes, although you can start to drink many decoctions after 15 minutes if desired.

3. **Using a mesh strainer or cheesecloth (or both), pour off the liquid from the herb, strain, and cool.** If you're ready to drink it, just ladle straight out of the pot. If you want to save some for later, let the decoction cool down for at least 10 minutes before pouring the liquid into a heatproof quart jar for storage. The jar will be extremely hot so don't touch it with your bare hands and wait till it is cool enough to touch before moving it to the refrigerator. There, decoctions will keep for 3 days and up to a week.

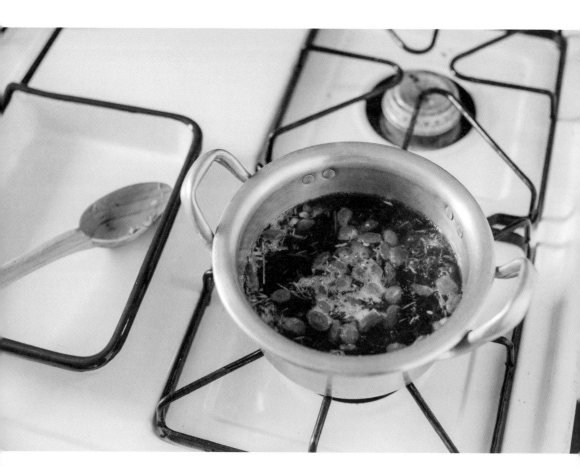

COMBINING DECOCTING AND INFUSING

What do you do if some of your chosen herbs need decocting and some need infusing? Don't panic! There is a solution for this predicament. Begin with the herbs you want to decoct, following the steps above. When you get to the part where you strain and cool, instead pour the decoction (herbs and all) into a 2-quart jar filled with the herbs you want to infuse. Cap lightly and proceed as you would for an infusion. In 4 to 12 hours you'll have your super-powered incoction or defusion or whatever you want to call your drink.

WHICH PLANTS IN THIS BOOK SHOULD I DECOCT?

Cinnamon

Dandelion root

Dried ginger root

Elderberries

Hawthorn berries

CLASSIC DECOCTION COMBINATIONS

Cinnamon stick or chips + dandelion root + chicory root (coffee replacement)

Dandelion root + burdock root + cacao nibs (skin and liver support)

Rose hips + hawthorn berries + vanilla bean (uplifting heart helper)

Shiitake + garlic + ginger (winter tonic)

Hawthorn berries + goji berry + cinnamon (hydrating vitamin boost)

Cinnamon + dandelion root + cardamom + clove (spring renewal)

Cacao + reishi + cinnamon (stress-fighting hot chocolate)

Elderberry + ginger (warming immune support)

Elderberry + rosehips (cooling immune support)

Fennel + dandelion root + ginger (digestive aid)

Herbal Syrup

An herbal syrup is basically an infused simple syrup (sweetener and water). Syrups, like honeys, are great medicines when attempting to please children or people with sensitive palates. Many herbs that we use in syrups are already tasty, so adding sweetener only accentuates what is already there to love. Adding sugar to something remotely sweet is like adding salt to something remotely savory: it brings out the flavor more.

Syrups are also incredibly versatile—they are delicious in tea, drizzled atop butter on baked goods, and over ice cream. Syrups are a great way to get your medicine and also an easy way to make things that are "bad for us" a little bit healthier! It's a convenient half-truth, but it works for me. And who wouldn't love elderberry syrup on vanilla ice cream? **Makes about 2 cups**.

1 cup dried herb(s) of choice (double for fresh)

2½ cups water

½ to 2 cups raw brown sugar or honey (see Which Sweetener Should I Choose? on page 79)

1 oz brandy or tincture per cup of syrup (optional)

1. **Prepare an infusion, a decoction, or a combination of the two (depending on the herbs you've chosen)** in a 2-quart saucepan. Your ratio of plant matter to water will be 1 cup of herb to 2½ cups of liquid. Infuse or decoct, uncovered, for 30 to 40 minutes; if you are decocting and infusing, decoct first for 20 then infuse for 20.

2. **Using a mesh strainer or cheesecloth (or both),** strain off the liquid from the herb and measure the reduction. If it has not reduced by half then return the liquid to the saucepan, and on a very low simmer reduce the total liquid volume to about half the original amount (1 cup).

3. **Add your sweetener.** If you want a thick syrup then use sugar, which you **can add directly** to the pan, keeping it over very low heat until dissolved. If you're using honey remove the reduction from the stovetop and then add the sweetener. Do the "back of the spoon" test: dip a spoon in the syrup, run your finger down the middle of the back of the spoon, and if the syrup stays in place you've achieved a thick syrup consistency.

4. **Remove the saucepan from the heat and add brandy or a tincture, if desired.** You could add brandy if you're making a cough syrup, or some other tincture relevant to your syrup. The alcohol will extend the shelf life of the syrup as well as serve as a warming relaxant.

5. **Pour the syrup into a glass pint jar, label, and store in the refrigerator.** Herbal syrups last at least 3 months in the refrigerator, usually longer.

WHICH SWEETENER SHOULD I CHOOSE?

I hate to break it to you but using raw sugar in a syrup doesn't necessarily mean it's good for you. Raw sugar is less refined than white sugar, so the presence of molasses gives it that brown hue. But because the percentage of molasses is very small, the presence of good-for-you things like iron and minerals is negligible.

Honey contains lots of good-for-you things, but it still contains sugar! Honey is rich in water-soluble vitamins (things like vitamin C that don't live in the body and need to be replaced every day), essential amino acids (those required by all vertebrates that our cells cannot synthesize), minerals like calcium, potassium, and magnesium, plus it's high in antioxidants. Why not add it to a burdock root syrup?

How much sweetener you use depends on what kind of sweetener, how much sweet you want, and how long you want your syrup to stay good. If you're using honey, a 1:1 liquid to sweetener ratio will stabilize the syrup for at least a month and up to 6 in the refrigerator, but that might be too sweet for some people. Using less sweetener just means it might not last as long, but when prepared in smaller amounts and stored in the refrigerator this shouldn't be a problem.

Herbal Oil Two Ways

An herbal oil is an extraction of an herb into a base oil. These are oils we use externally on our body, face, or hair, made from oils that we cook and eat with every day (think olive oil). Like tea, the process of making an herbal oil is not only relaxing but provides a luxurious end result as well. How does it feel to spend 3 minutes lovingly nourishing your skin and hair? What would 10 minutes feel like? What does it mean to pay attention to all the parts of ourselves and notice that they function together on one body? Each part deserves to be noticed and loved. Time spent making and applying an herbal oil can be a key part of that practice.

How to Make an Herbal Oil

My favorite two ways to make an herbal oil are the solar and double-boiler methods:

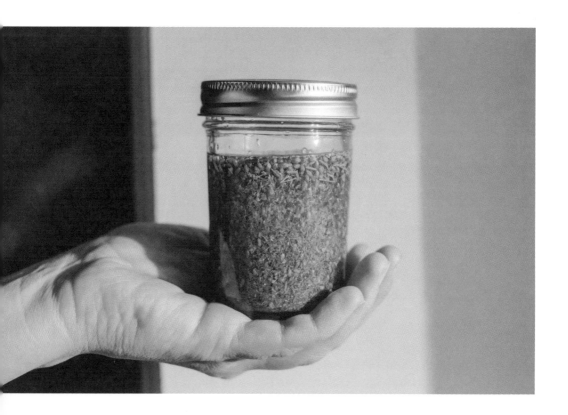

Solar Method

I recommend using dried herbs for this method of making an herbal oil. If you really want to use fresh herbs, then use the double-boiler method. **Makes about 1 cup**.

1 cup dried herb of choice, roughly chopped before measuring

1½ cups oil of choice

5 to 10 drops of essential oil (optional)

½ teaspoon vitamin E oil (optional)

1. **Add the herbs to a glass pint jar** (the herbs will fill the jar about two-thirds of the way, leaving 1 to 3 inches of space above your herbs).

2. **Add the oil to the jar.** Stir to make sure that the herbs are completely coated in oil and the oil covers the herbs by at least 1 inch.

3. **Cover the mouth of the jar with a small square of waxed paper, cap tightly, and label.** I like to put the label for oils on the top of the jar, as oil will tend to leak out no matter how tightly you screw on the lid. Shake thoroughly. Wipe up any oil that's snuck out and put the jar on top of a small plate or plastic lid in direct sunlight.

4. **Shake the jar daily over 2 to 3 weeks.**

5. **Strain.** Lay a piece of cheesecloth over a fine-mesh strainer and pour the oil into a clean, dry jar. As the herbs fall into the strainer, I like to move the squeezed-out herbs into my compost bin little by little rather than trying to handle a huge clump of oily herbs at the end.

6. **Add any additional oils, update your label, and store.** Now's the time to add essential oils to your infused oil! Maybe a little orange and geranium to that calendula-infused face oil, or some rosemary to your arnica sore muscle massage oil. Vitamin E oil, a powerful oil that works well in partnership with other oils, will extend the shelf life of your herbal oil. Do note that vitamin E can cause skin outbreaks on some people, so test a small spot on your skin first.

7. **Your herbal oil will keep for a year at room temperature.** Even though the bathroom may seem like a good place to store face, body, and hair oil, over time a hot, humid environment might cause it to spoil quickly. A better idea is to keep large batches in cool, dry places (I keep mine in my kitchen) and store smaller 1-ounce bottles for daily use in the bathroom. This limits the chance of water sneaking in so your oils will last longer.

Double-Boiler Method

I prefer the solar method for oil making in almost all circumstances except for specific plants that require they be prepared fresh (more on that later) and when I'm pressed for time. While the solar method can take up to 4 weeks, the double-boiler method means I can have my oil in a matter of hours! It only requires that I be present to replenish the water in the bottom pot and make sure my herbs don't fry.

Makes about 1 cup.

1 cup dried herbs of choice, or 2 cups finely chopped fresh herbs

1½ cups oil of choice

5 to 10 drops essential oil (optional)

½ teaspoon vitamin E oil (optional)

1. If using fresh herbs, wilt your plants for at least 24 hours before beginning. Herbs like St. John's wort, chickweed, and jewelweed make the best oil when fresh, but pre-wilting overnight is still a good idea. Any water left in the prepared oil will increase the likelihood of spoilage: the less water you start with, the less you have to cook off. When using fresh herbs, ending up with more oil than the amount you started with could indicate that some water remains in your oil.

2. **Fill the bottom pot of a double boiler or saucepan with water.** Make sure the water doesn't touch the bottom of the top pot or the glass bowl as that will overheat the oil and the herb.

3. **Add the herbs to the double boiler or glass bowl set atop the saucepan (but not in contact with the water) and cover with the oil.** The oil should cover the herbs completely.

4. **Simmer for 1 to 8 hours,** keeping the temperature between 95°F and 110°F; we are going for extraction, not fried herbs to garnish your dinner. If you prefer to use a thermometer to gauge the temperature, feel free. Remove from the heat and let the mixture cool.

5. **Strain.** Lay a piece of cheesecloth over a fine-mesh strainer and pour the oil into a clean, dry jar. As the herbs fall into the strainer, I like to move the squeezed-out herbs into my compost bin little by little rather than trying to handle a huge clump of oily herbs at the end. If using fresh herbs you might find 3 to 7 days after making it that some leftover watery gunk accumulated on the bottom of the jar. If so, carefully pour off the oil into a new, clean jar and discard the leftover water and sediment.

6. **Add any additional oils, label your jar, and store.** Now's the time to add essential oils to your infused oil, if you desire! Maybe a little orange and geranium to that calendula-infused face oil, or some rosemary to your arnica sore-muscle massage oil. Vitamin E oil, a powerful oil that works well in partnership with other oils, will extend the shelf life of your herbal oil. Do note that vitamin E can cause skin outbreaks on some people, so test a small spot on your skin first.

7. **Your herbal oil will keep for a year at room temperature.** Even though the bathroom may seem like a good place to store face, body, and hair oil, a hot, humid environment might cause it to spoil quickly. A better idea is to keep large batches in cool, dry places (I keep mine in my kitchen) and store smaller 1-ounce bottles for daily use in the bathroom. This limits the chance of water sneaking in so your oils will last longer.

WHAT KIND OF OIL SHOULD I USE?

For culinary oils, I love olive oil. My favorite is an infused rosemary oil that I coat a whole chicken with before putting it in the oven. I'm on the dry side, so I also love using olive oil for my skin. I don't mind the slight hint of olives and my skin really drinks it up. If you tend not to experience dryness then you might like a lighter oil; avocado or sesame oil are great for hair and skin. For my face, I prefer jojoba oil with a little vitamin E.

Make small amounts using different oils of the same herb when you're starting out so you can test what's right for you! In terms of quality, buy the best you can afford. You can purchase most of these oils at the grocery store, so be sure to read the labels carefully. Remember that putting oil on your skin is like giving your body a drink from the outside, so choose wisely.

HOW DO I KNOW IF MY OIL IS BAD?

When an oil is off it can smell bitter, metallic, soapy, or cheesy. This can happen to the end product if water was present when you made the oil. I know you spent all that time shaking your oil jar or giving your herbs a warm oil bath, lovingly stirring and patiently waiting for the time when you could slather it all over your thirsty skin, but you're just going to have to throw that rancid stuff away. Your skin is your largest organ. It's part of you, it absorbs *everything*, including bad stuff, so give yourself a break, cut your losses, and begin again.

WHICH HERBS ARE BEST FOR OILS?

Aerial (aboveground) parts of herbs are most commonly used in herbal oils, but below ground plants are not off limits. You can use herbs that soothe sensitive skin or provide relief after a bug bite like chamomile, calendula, or plantain; herbs that deliver added moisture like chickweed or soothe sore muscles like rosemary, arnica, and St. John's wort; herbs for your ears like garlic and mullein; or herbs to calm like lavender and rose.

SO, ARE THESE ESSENTIAL OILS?

Nope! Essential oils are volatile, which means they evaporate when exposed to air, which is why we can smell them! Essential oils come from plant tissue and can be made by pressing a plant (like oregano oil or citrus oils), steaming it in a still (like lavender oil), or synthetically with chemical solvents. Vegetable oils like olive oil, sesame oil, and almond oil are non-volatile, meaning they don't evaporate, because they are high in fat.

WHICH ESSENTIAL OILS SHOULD I BUY?

Working with essential oils originated sometime between 980 and 1037 in Persia by a man named Ibn Sina, commonly known by his westernized name Avicenna. By all accounts, Ibn Sina was basically a genius: nicknamed the "prince of physicians," he united Greek and Arab medical practices, outlined specific procedures for trauma, recorded medicinal recipes, and perfected the distillation process of essential oils. The practice of working with essential oils in a therapeutic setting was coined "aromatherapy" by the French perfumer and chemist René Gattefossé in 1937. In recent years, the essential oil market has exploded and it can be overwhelming to navigate. How can you be sure the company you buy from prioritizes the well-being of plants, humans, and the planet?

Look for the following information on the essential oil label: plant common name, Latin name (genus and species), where the plant comes from (what country), which part of the plant they used, how the plant was processed (pressing, distillation, or synthetically), and how it was grown (organic, non-GMO, wild-crafted, etc.). What's important to you will determine which categories you want to see represented on the label. If you're unable to find information about a company's growing or labor practices, choose another one that makes that information available and consider that the more expensive price tag might be worth it. While it can be tempting to buy cheap essential oil, this is generally an indication that best practices aren't being followed. To put it into perspective: It takes 242,000 rose petals to make 5 milliliters of rose oil. It takes 3 pounds of lavender to produce 15 milliliters of lavender essential oil. That's *a lot* of plant. Dousing yourself in essential oil is not the goal. A little essential oil goes a long way and in many cases you are making at least a year's investment, sometimes more! Still stressed about the price? A great way to offset the financial and environmental burden is to form an essential oil collective with friends. You can all gather to share resources and make stuff together. The more the merrier.

Salve

A salve is what is commonly known as an ointment: an oily, semi-solid, topical preparation for the skin. Salves, like tinctures, are excellent medicines on the go—you can keep them in your backpack, purse, canvas bag, pocket, and first aid kit. Choose shallow containers with screw-top lids. You will inevitably forget the salve someplace warm and it will melt and leak out a bit. Your chances of saving your upholstery, clothes, or bag are always improved with a screw-top lid. By storing the salve in multiple containers you can give them as gifts to friends or squirrel them away in different parts of your house, apartment, and workplace. Then you have a salve everywhere you go.

Salves and oils are great medicines for cuts and burns that are already on their way toward healing because they lock stuff in and keep stuff out. If you have a fresh burn, avoid applying oil or salve to the area because this traps the heat that your body needs to expel in order to heal. Honey is a great band-aid for a fresh burn (as long as it doesn't require professional medical attention) because it cools the unbearable sensation of a lingering burn, keeps the area moist, and fights infection with its antimicrobial properties.

As with honey and oil, buy the best-quality beeswax you can afford (you can use a block or beads/pellets). If you want to make a vegan salve, you can use carnauba wax instead of beeswax. **Makes about 2 cups.**

SPECIAL EQUIPMENT:
SHALLOW GLASS
OR TIN STORAGE
CONTAINERS WITH
SCREW-TOP LIDS

1 cup herbal oil
(page 80)

1 cup grated beeswax
or in pellet/bead
form

½ teaspoon (roughly
50 drops) essential
oil or perfume
(optional)

1. **Put a small metal spoon in the freezer.**

2. **Fill the bottom pot of a double boiler or saucepan with water.** Make sure the water doesn't touch the bottom of the pot or the top of the glass bowl, which would overheat the oil and the herb.

3. **Combine the herbal oil and beeswax in the top pot of your double boiler or your glass bowl.** Turn the heat to low and stir often to dissolve the beeswax into the oil as it warms, between 10 and 15 minutes.

4. **Turn the heat off and test the consistency of your salve.** Take your metal spoon from the freezer, dip it into the salve, and set it back in the freezer on a plate. After 5 minutes check how it has set up; this is a simulation of the consistency of your final salve. If you want a

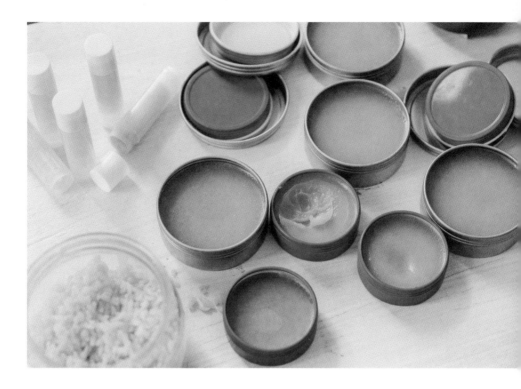

harder salve, add a little more beeswax; for a softer salve, add more oil. If the salve in your double boiler or bowl set up while you were testing it, just turn the heat on low to gently rewarm the salve.

5. **Add essential oil or perfume, if desired.** If you want to blend different scents then do so before adding it to the salve. Do your experimenting in a glass shot glass or small bowl, because essential oils will break down certain plastics over time.

6. **Immediately pour the salve into storage containers.** The salve will settle as it cools which means it will be slightly concave. Let it cool and set a bit, and then rewarm what's left in your pot and top off the salve in the container.

7. **Label the top of the container with the ingredients and date.** Salves will keep for several months in a cool dark place out of direct sunlight and extreme heat.

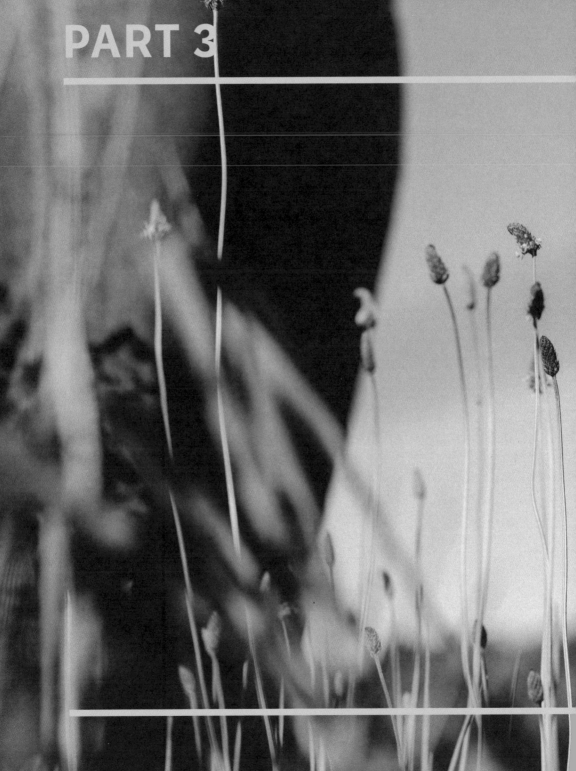

PART 3

YOUR
HERBAL
ARSENAL

It's great to read about plants, but it's even better to actually drink them, eat them, and put them on your body! We have arrived at the plants that can make a great foundation to your medicinal arsenal. If you don't take the time to *really* know plants, then you'll never know which ones you need and you'll definitely never know which ones other people might need. Here are profiles of twenty-one plants that grow in close proximity to humans. Some are native and others are not. Some are wild while others have become cornerstones of pollinator gardens, highway median landscaping, and clever invaders of cracks in parking lots and window boxes. All of them can be found in cities, most growing wild in parks and on city blocks, while others can be found at farmers markets, grocery stores, and bodegas. Among them you'll find a nutritive antidote to spring allergies, tiny berries packed with vitamin C, an instant latex-free band-aid, and so much more.

How to Understand Plant Profiles

Each plant profile communicates my experience with the plant: what I love about it, how I look for it, the ways I work with it. This is not an exhaustive *materia medica* of every plant. You will not love every plant I love. My hope is that you find your own ways of connecting and working with plants. You will develop your own language for describing how each feels in and on your body. Perhaps you'll crave a cooling chickweed salve as your radiators blast heat and zap your apartment of all available moisture. Or after reading an upsetting story in the newspaper you'll reach impulsively for rose petals and linden to make a quick cup of tea that feels like a comforting embrace. In order to help you do that I've identified some key characteristics of each plant. The next page shows a sample of the framework that each profile follows and an explanation of what to expect in each subheading.

Common Name

This is how the plant is referred to colloquially in my region in the United States. In general there is more than one common name for a plant. If you think or hear of other common names, add them to the entry!

Latin Name

The Latin binomial name is standardized, which means that no matter where you are in the world you can identify a plant by its Latin name.

Reach for this when	The circumstances and experiences to which the plant is best suited
Sensation	How the plant feels in our bodies
Flavors	How the plant tastes
Where it lives	Where you might find the plant
Gather this	The ingestible or applicable parts of the plant
Super strengths	A list of generally accepted "plant actions" (see page 32 for definitions)

WHY I'M IN LOVE

All the best bits, in my opinion! These are generally drawn from precious *aha* moments with the plant. As you familiarize yourself with a plant you will also have these experiences—write these moments down. I've learned a lot from reading about and listening to more experienced herbalists' study and understanding of a plant. At this point in time we have access to accumulated and emerging knowledge from all over the world and from many cultures. These records are invaluable as we embark on a lifetime of botanical discovery. Of equal value are quiet moments at home with a cup of tea, a realization in the shower, and even a dream in which a plant appears to you. These are the places where you move from intellectualizing a plant to beginning to understand where to embody its actions, build affection for it, and decide to protect it.

WHAT IT DOES BEST

An elaboration on the actions described in "Reach for this when" and a more detailed description of the circumstances for which the plant is best suited.

HOW IT GROWS

Physical characteristics of the plant and a more detailed description of its preferred habitat.

TO RECAP

Key takeaways

You should feel encouraged to keep your own notes in the plant profiles. Yes, in this book. Write all over everything, highlight, and draw. You will better understand and remember the plants if you can make your own imprint of your experience with them. Try not to be afraid or embarrassed to be your own expert! Move confidently in your partnership with plants. They are eager to have you on their team—if you show up for them, they'll surely show up for you.

A NOTE ABOUT NATIVE PLANTS

Many of our common weeds in the United States were either brought here intentionally or found their way stuck to the soles of shoes or clinging to a piece of luggage. As modern people with a perspective on history, we can make choices today that steward and support native plants so that they may thrive for the native populations that need them most. As a person of Western European descent, day to day I work primarily with the plants that came from the part of the world that my ancestors did, not because they're better but because they're part of my history and are invasive. For this reason, most of the plants in this section are of that tradition, with a few exceptions. White pine is one of the few plants in this book that is indigenous to the United States. If you are like me and are not only not indigenous to this country, but also are of colonizer heritage, I would encourage you to consider the impact of wild-crafting any plant that holds special meaning for indigenous populations.

American Elderberry

Sambucus canadensis

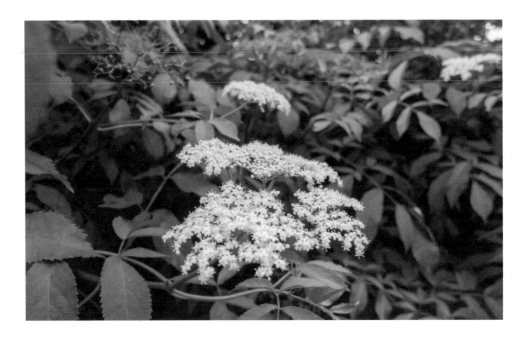

Reach for this when	It's flu season, during times of transition or tension
Sensation	Flowers: cool, dry Berries: relaxing, stimulating, cooling, moistening
Flavors	Flowers: sweet, musky lemon Berries: sweet, tannic
Where it lives	On the edge—bordering walking paths, growing next to the multiuse asphalt, squeezed between a fence and a driveway
Gather this	Flowers and berries (avoid bark and leaves which can be laxative and toxic in high-enough doses)
Super strengths	Alterative, sedative, stimulant, expectorant, diuretic, astringent, demulcent, emollient, laxative, diaphoretic, nervine, tonic, relaxant, anti-inflammatory

WHY I'M IN LOVE

In the spring I like to ride my bike the long way home: meandering on the bridge over the East River, past the overgrown Navy Yard, and up a steady hill to Prospect Park. My bike ride is an effective form of decompressing: it shuttles blood through my heavy legs (I stand all day at work, every day) and eases the transition from work to home. I can feel the stress and responsibility fall away the further I peddle from Manhattan, the last of it melting off as I scan the horizon for puffs of white elder flowers and sail down the hill toward the lake. Elder is a particularly helpful plant for transitions: the flowers for when we need help moving forward, the berries for when we're on the edge of illness and need help moving back to health.

WHAT IT DOES BEST

Every fall my aunt saves the berries from the elder that hangs over her driveway and freezes them for me. When I go up north to visit I pack them in my luggage and take them home to make a delicious, immune-strengthening syrup. Elderberry is perhaps best known for fighting the flu as it directly inhibits the action of the flu virus, regardless of the strain, and reduces the symptoms and length of sickness. For this reason elderberry is an effective medicine to take even if you got your seasonal flu vaccine: flu shots only vaccinate against specific strains, and the virus is skilled at mutating. Elderberry attacks all flu strains even as they evolve to skillfully escape destruction. It's also effective against other types of illness. I take a spoonful anytime the familiar signs of sluggish sickness arise and I find myself telling people that I'm "fighting something off," like when I can't drink enough water to keep my lips from chapping, my body feels lethargic, or seven o'clock feels like a perfectly reasonable bedtime. Elderberry is high in vitamin C, effectively anti-inflammatory, and appropriate for almost any constitution. The sweet syrup is at once medicinal and comforting.

Mythology around the elder tree identifies it as a symbol of sorrow and death. It grows on the edge of the wild and the cultivated, occupying a liminal space. It can be helpful as an ally when we are teetering on the brink of acceptance. Physically it can help us find balance by simultaneously stimulating and sedating. It relaxes mental and muscular gripping, but also releases heat and tension. The flowers taken as a tea can help to encourage a productive fever and ease us to sleep.

HOW IT GROWS

The American elder is a sprawling shrub that can grow up to 10 feet tall, sometimes taller. It likes moist soil along fences, borders, and paths. Small, white flowers bloom in May and taper off toward the end of June (depending on how hot the summer is). The flowers grow in a sprawling manner botanically known as a cyme: an arrangement of flowers in which the central flowers open first. Clusters of berries (known as drupes) ripen in the fall. They are deep purple and make a magenta-colored juice.

Elder is great for emotional and physical vulnerability. It can shore up our immune system when we are most vulnerable in winter. Whether it's coming home from work or coming out of a relationship, elder is appropriate for all the liminal spaces where we need support and release, helping us to move through and carry on.

Elderflower Toner

I like to use the stuff I make to establish routines, marking consistent moments in the day reserved for checking in and taking care of myself. Elderflower is toning to our skin, at once astringent and emollient. Combined with calendula and chamomile flowers, you can make a soothing toner in no time. **Makes about 1 cup.**

1 cup witch hazel

1 tablespoon dried elderflower

1½ teaspoons dried calendula flowers

1½ teaspoons dried chamomile flowers

1 teaspoon glycerin (optional)

Combine the witch hazel, elderflower, calendula, and chamomile in a glass pint jar, cap, and label with the date. Place in a cool spot out of direct sunlight. Shake the jar every couple of days over the next month. Strain off the herbs and compost them. If your skin is dry, you can add the glycerin to your toner. Transfer your toner to a spray bottle or store in a bottle with a screw cap and use a cotton ball to apply after washing your face.

Elderberry Syrup

I look forward to making elderberry syrup every fall as we prepare for the transition to winter. I slowly clean the berries from the delicate stems and gather all the other plants to make a remedy for winter colds and flus. I keep my syrup in the fridge because I like how it tastes cool. I take 1 tablespoon at the first sign of sickness. Pro tip: it also makes an excellent addition to a cold-weather bowl of ice cream. **Makes 1 cup.**

½ cup dried elderberries

¼ cup dried orange peel

2 tablespoons cinnamon chips

2 tablespoons chopped dried ginger root

2½ cups water

½ cup honey

Combine the elderberries, orange peel, cinnamon, ginger, and water in a small saucepan, turn the heat to medium and bring to a simmer for 5 to 7 minutes. Turn down to low and simmer for 30 to 40 minutes partially covered. Strain into a liquid measuring cup, being sure to press the plants into the mesh strainer or cheesecloth to squeeze out all the liquid. You should have about 1 cup of liquid; if you have more than 1 cup, return the liquid to the stove and let it reduce on low heat a little longer. Remove from the heat and stir in the honey until it dissolves. Store in a glass bottle with a tight-fitting lid. I keep my syrup in the refrigerator where it will last up to a year.

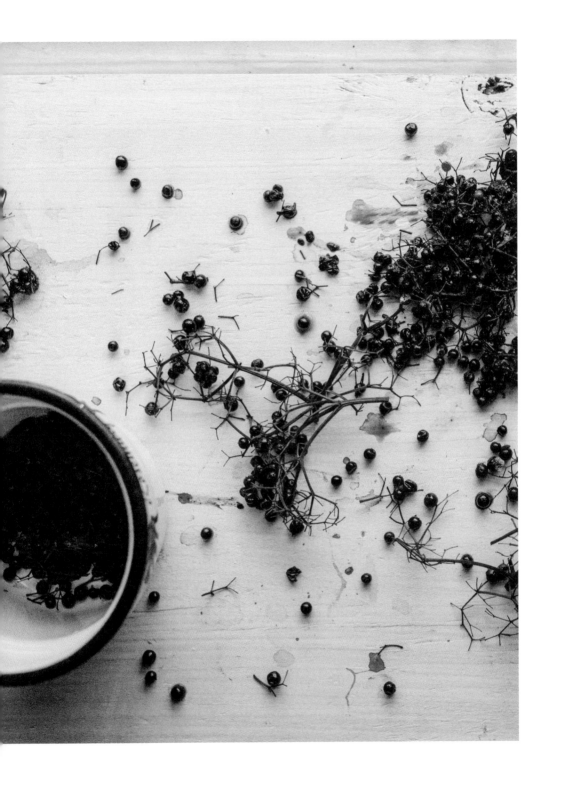

Catnip

Nepeta cataria

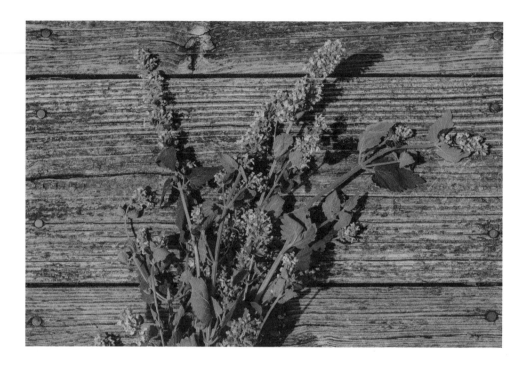

Reach for this when	You need to calm your stomach, induce sweating to release fever, soothe mild menstrual pain
Sensation	Cooling, moistening
Flavors	Bitter, minty, lemony
Where it lives	Full sun with some afternoon shade, in gardens and as city plants in parks, bordering walking paths and vehicles lanes
Gather this	Leaves, flowers
Super strengths	Antispasmodic, relaxant, diaphoretic, slightly emmenagogic, carminative

WHY I'M IN LOVE

Catnip is all over my city: in the gardens bordering the large houses just outside my neighborhood, in the medians that divide larger avenues, in my window, and at the farmers market. There is always a lot and it is generally perky: sturdy, upright, sprawling a bit. It says a certain something to have so much of one plant in such a bananas city.

WHAT IT DOES BEST

While catnip relaxes, it is also gently stimulating. It is helpful in places where we encounter obstacles and blockages. I don't think it's a coincidence that I always encounter catnip where paths meet, especially in the city when bicycle, walking, and motorized vehicle lanes come to a head. It's my tendency to meet these moments of congestion or decision with principled resoluteness and a tightness of determination. The circumstance necessitates a certain amount of assertion in order to stay alert and not get run over, but it's a fine line between asserting yourself and aggression. Catnip's ability to stimulate and soothe simultaneously means that we remain on-point while we calm down: it grants us a clarity to discern quickly without falling into a frenzy. Catnip calms us in all the places where we feel like we can't get a grip and want to lash out. In our bodies, catnip does something similar in offering release through calming actions. It dispels gas in our digestive system, gently moves a stalled menstrual cycle, and eases tight headaches. All of these things point to an overall relaxing action in our bodies and

minds. As it cools, it opens, offering pathways that alleviate and allow for space to be made.

HOW IT GROWS

Catnip thrives in dry soils and is tolerant of drought and pollution. It's forgiving and generous, a great city plant for the person who forgets they have plants. If you're skilled at remembering to water your plants then it will appreciate your thoughtfulness by rewarding you with an abundance of minty leaves beginning in early spring and tiny white and purplish flowers in late summer. There are a few different varieties: Cat*mint* is common in the Northeast and it grows not quite as high as catnip and its flowers are a deeper purple. All varieties are perennial, so you can expect it year after year.

TO RECAP

Whether it's an overtired baby wailing at bedtime or the adult who just wants to crumble because it's Monday and they have to go to work again, a cup of catnip tea is like the heavy, comforting lower back rub that says "I know, it's ok. You don't have to be so tough." It can help us relax into our feelings and then give us the gentle stimulation to move through them so we can do what we have to do: go to sleep or go to work with more ease and comfort.

Smoking Blend

Occasionally smoking herbs can offer a quiet moment of reflection and peace. It can help the responsibilities and worry of the day fall away as you move into time at home or with friends and in the evening as part of a before-bed routine. That being said, we are still inhaling smoke and smoking habitually is bad for your lungs and overall health. However, if you're trying to quit smoking tobacco cigarettes, rolling your own cigarettes and slowly phasing out the tobacco can be a great way to quit. Calming herbs like catnip are especially helpful for the anxiety that accompanies withdrawal and cravings. **Makes about ¼ cup of blend.**

2 tablespoons dried mullein leaf

1 tablespoon dried raspberry leaf

½ tablespoon dried catnip leaf

Sprinkling of dried lavender flowers

Rolling papers

Combine the mullein, raspberry, and catnip in a bowl and sprinkle with the lavender. Rub the herbs between your fingers so that they get fuzzy and stick together. The smoking blend will store better in an airtight container (a tin or glass jar with a screw-top lid) than as pre-rolled cigarettes. Before rolling an herbal cigarette you may need to add a drop of water to the mixture so that it stays together better while you roll it and smokes more smoothly.

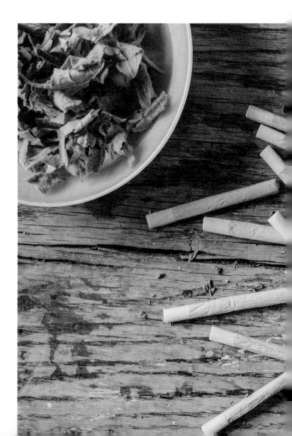

Butterfly Tea Blend

Catnip is perfect for anyone who reports butterflies in their stomach due to nervousness or anxiety. This is a handy tea to have at home and is appropriate to drink day or night. **Makes 2 cups.**

1 cup dried catnip leaves and flowers
½ cup dried fennel seed
½ cup dried chamomile flowers

Combine the herbs in a glass pint jar. To make tea for one, boil 1 cup of water, remove from the heat, and allow it to sit as you measure and prepare your serving. Steep 2 tablespoons of the blend in a lidded container (to keep the volatile oils from escaping) for 10 minutes and then strain. Sip and feel the butterflies fly away.

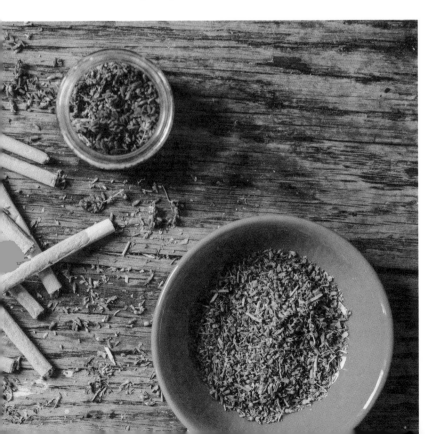

Cinnamon

Cinnamomum zeylanicum (Ceylon cinnamon),
C. cassia (cassia cinnamon)

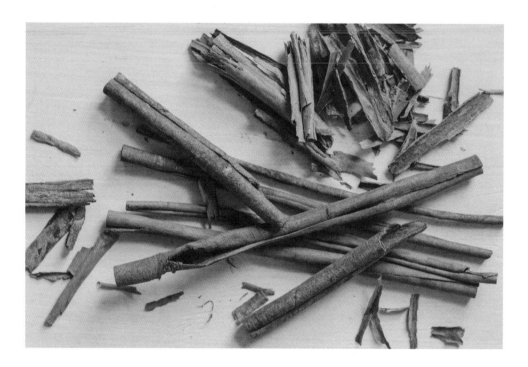

Reach for this when	You're eating something sweet, you need help getting your digestion or circulation going, you've been experiencing tummy trouble or congestion in your lungs
Sensation	Warming, drying
Flavors	Spicy, sweet
Where it lives	Mostly on plantations in the tropics with climates that support rainforests
Gather this	Leaf, bark (technically the inner bark)
Super strengths	Stimulant, demulcent, carminative, nutritive, tonic, stomachic, antimicrobial, diaphoretic, astringent, anodyne

WHY I'M IN LOVE

When I cooked in restaurants I worked the line with a guy from France who detested cinnamon. If anyone dared to present a family meal dessert with cinnamon he made no effort at hiding his disgust. "Americans," he'd say shaking his head, "always with the fucking cinnamon and always too much." And this is precisely what I love about cinnamon—it is everywhere. Adorning the soft peaks of whipped cream atop autumn's long anticipated and equally loathed pumpkin spice lattes, then mixed with nutmeg and sprinkled on eggnog lattes once the snow hits. In and on top of snickerdoodles, oatmeal raisin cookies, rice pudding, bread pudding, cinnamon rolls. And what about toast? In New York, with a population from all over the world, I find cinnamon in the Jewish, Arab, Mexican, and West Indian bakeries of my neighborhood; in the spice blends at the Korean, Chinese, and Indian Markets; and even the vegan spot on the corner that doesn't do dairy. All to say there's no such thing as too much cinnamon, in my opinion.

WHAT IT DOES BEST

Besides managing to be among the world's most popular spices, cinnamon is probably most famous for calming blood sugar spikes. Some studies show it may do so by lowering insulin resistance. Since medieval times (at least) people have identified the usefulness of combining cinnamon and sugar. Personally, I find I can combat some of the draining effects of overindulging in sugar at the holidays by brewing a strong cup of cinnamon tea or generously sprinkling some of the ground spice into my tea or coffee: the spike that sends me into a tizzy is calmed and I don't come crashing to a halt 30 minutes later.

Cinnamon also works as a stimulant internally and when applied topically. If you've ever stupidly tried to pull the plastic part out of an essential oil bottle with your teeth and splashed cinnamon essential oil all over your upper lip then you might know what I'm talking about. When your friend sees you 25 minutes later and exclaims "I think you're having an allergic reaction!" You can calmly tell her, "It's ok, I'm just locally stimulating my upper lip." Which might be helpful, in *extremely* low dose applications, if you've been outside working in the cold or intend to spend the day hitting the slopes. Internally a strong tea or powdered cinnamon mixed with honey is among my go-to remedies for abdominal cramps from menstruation and my favorite remedy for painful diarrhea, as it increases circulation and moves gas along.

HOW IT GROWS

This beautiful tropical tree is prized for its edible bark. The only place you'll be gathering cinnamon is in places like Sri Lanka, Ceylon, cinnamon's native home, or in your fancy greenhouse that resembles a lush, wet, tropical forest. Otherwise you're likely reaching for it in the baking aisle at your grocery store. While there are over 250 varieties of cinnamon worldwide, the most popular variety I see is cassia though I do come across Ceylon and Korintje.

TO RECAP

If it's confusing to think of cinnamon as both moistening and drying, here's a challenge to try. If you put a teaspoon of cinnamon powder in a glass of water it will absorb the water and carry that into your body where it can be easily absorbed. But if you put the cinnamon powder in your mouth it will suck up all the moisture in there and make it impossible to swallow. Cinnamon is a great example of the complexities of plant actions! It is abundant and widely available. It adorns that which it controls: the sugar that threatens to send our bodies crashing or worse into chronic illness. At once comforting and strongly medicinal, it's no wonder cinnamon has a place in so many cultures.

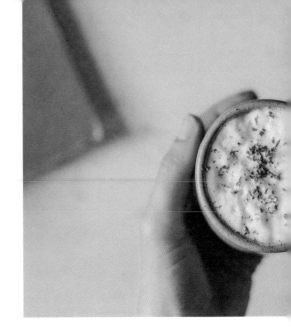

Cinnamon Latte

This is the perfect drink for a Sunday afternoon at home with a book on a cool autumn day. Its mild sweetness is a good swap for that four o'clock nudge from a chocolate chip cookie: comforting, warming, and gently stimulating. **Makes 2 drinks.**

One 3-inch cinnamon stick

2 cardamom pods

½ teaspoon dried ginger

2 black peppercorns

2 cups milk of your choice

2 teaspoons honey

Cinnamon powder and whole nutmeg
(optional)

Wrap the cinnamon stick, cardamom, ginger, and peppercorns in a piece of cheesecloth and tie it off with a piece of kitchen twine. Add the herb bundle and milk to a small saucepan and heat over medium-low until tiny bubbles form around the edge of the pan. Stir often, keeping the milk warm and under a simmer, for 5 minutes. Use a slotted spoon to lift the bundle out of the milk and into your compost. Add the honey if desired and whisk vigorously to foam the herbal milk. Or if you're lazy like me, put the honey in a blender, pour the milk over it and buzz on low to foam the milk. Finish with a dusting of cinnamon and a grating of nutmeg if you like.

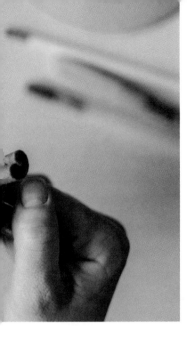

Body Scrub

In drier climates and seasons our bodies could do with a little exfoliating. You can make a simple enlivening scrub from ingredients you probably already have lying around in your kitchen! If you prefer a finer scrub, use granulated sugar instead of turbinado. **Makes about 1 cup.**

¾ cup turbinado or granulated sugar

3 teaspoons cinnamon powder

¼ cup olive oil

3 tablespoons honey

Combine the sugar, cinnamon, oil, and honey in a bowl and stir well with a spatula. Store in a shallow wide plastic jar in your bathroom. When your feet, knees, or elbows get dry and flaky, put a little scrub on your forefinger and rub gently to exfoliate while you're bathing or showering. It's not even a big deal if you sneak a little taste.

WHAT'S THE DIFFERENCE?

Ceylon cinnamon is named for the country from which it originated, Sri Lanka, formerly Ceylon. It is commonly referred to as "true" or "real" cinnamon, which is a misnomer because the other cinnamons aren't any less real. It's mainly that the spectrum of flavor represented in cassia cinnamon is not as complex as in Ceylon. Cassia cinnamon is what we commonly find in grocery stores in the United States. Cassia contains a high concentration of cinnamaldehyde, which is the flavor in the essential oil that provides its characteristic sweetness.

IF YOU'RE ON BLOOD THINNERS

If you are on blood thinners, discuss with a professional how much cassia cinnamon is an appropriate therapeutic amount to consume. Cassia cinnamon also contains a high amount of coumarin, which when taken in large amounts acts as a blood-thinning agent. For this reason, many herbalists recommend Ceylon cinnamon for long-term therapeutic doses.

Chamomile

Matricaria recutita (German chamomile),
Chamaemelum nobile (Roman chamomile)

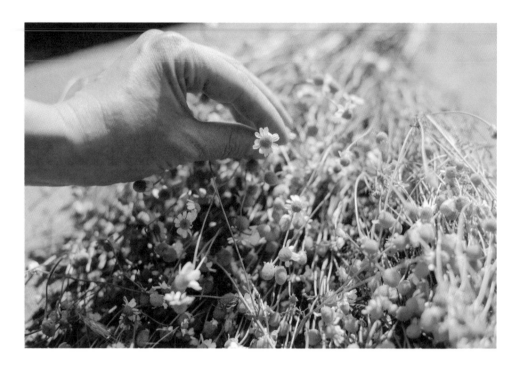

Reach for this when	You want to relax the nervous system, calm an aggressive fever, ease gas and bloating, soothe hot rashes or other skin conditions
Sensation	Mostly neutral
Flavors	Sweet like an apple with a bitter aftertaste
Where it lives	Sunny fields, grazed grasslands
Gather this	Flower tops hold stronger healing power, though tea made from the stems and leaves is still beneficial
Super strengths	Antispasmodic, anti-inflammatory, digestive, nervine, diaphoretic, carminative, anodyne, relaxant, bitter

WHY I'M IN LOVE

I like that I can count on chamomile to be pretty much anywhere: the grocery store, bodegas, and most importantly the airport. Not fresh of course, but dried and in a teabag. But when you're in a tight spot and feeling desperate, it can be just the thing to ease traveler's digestive issues like gas and bloating, even constipation. The inevitable bumps and hiccups of airborne travel can leave me feeling tired and cranky, like things just will never go my way. It can make a big difference to take a few minutes from whatever circumstances have me feeling like a helpless baby to track down a chamomile tea bag. Or better yet, just deploy the one stashed in my wallet next to my emergency mayonnaise packet.

WHAT IT DOES BEST

Chamomile is always appropriate in any situation with a lot of heat. In Peru a few years ago, I didn't wear enough sunscreen on the beach, near the equator at noon toward the end of their summer. I was super pink. Chamomile to the rescue! I picked up a healthy bunch at the market and made a compress, which relieved the pain and inflammation. It's also great for inflamed emotions: chamomile is the plant for the person who gets red-faced and veiny when mad.

Chamomile is also my favorite remedy for what I call the "Leave me alone! Don't leave me alone!" feelings. I can count on chamomile to relax and relieve the tension between this competing desire to be cared for and to turn people away. When feelings of anxiety spread to my digestive tract chamomile is in order. Ordinarily chamomile has a pleasantly floral-apple profile, but if you let it steep longer, the bitterness comes out. That bitter flavor can help relieve stagnant digestion triggered by feelings of nervousness or anxiety.

HOW IT GROWS

Chamomile prefers cooler summer climates, but I've seen it growing abundantly in sunny humid fields of pick-your-own strawberry farms in upstate New York. I haven't had luck with it as an indoor plant, but my friends with a roof garden report that their chamomile thrived up there. Roman chamomile is a perennial and slightly smaller than German chamomile: it grows about a foot high and has similar but smaller flowers. The Roman variety is identifiable by its fine and feathery foliage. German chamomile is an annual and grows to be twice as high as Roman chamomile. Its foliage is more fernlike and its flowers slightly larger and droopier. Though they look distinct, they have a similar healing personality.

TO RECAP

In my experience, chamomile is the most shrugged off of the medicinal plants. You'd think that its ubiquity would mean that more people would appreciate it, but the offer of chamomile tea is often met with a polite "no thank you" or worse "ugh, I hate warm hay water." I feel like that's because most people just haven't had a decent cup of chamomile tea. Yet. Who hates chamomile? People who need chamomile, that's who.

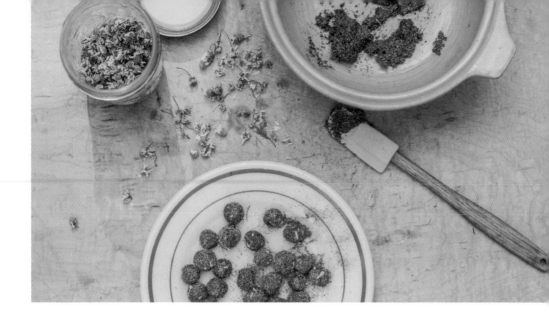

Calm-Me Pills

Herbal pills are great for people of all ages to make because it is an inherently messy and fun process. You can formulate your own blends to suit a variety of needs, applications, and circumstances. Like tinctures, they are portable. **Makes about 2 dozen pills.**

SPECIAL EQUIPMENT: DEHYDRATOR

1 tablespoon plus 1 teaspoon powdered chamomile, divided

2 teaspoons cacao powder, divided

2 teaspoons powdered lemon balm

1 teaspoon powdered angelica root

Pinch of nutmeg

Honey

Coconut oil (optional)

Combine 1 tablespoon of the chamomile, 1 teaspoon of the cacao, and the lemon balm, angelica, and nutmeg in a bowl. Drizzle in enough honey to form a stiff paste; it should be pliable and not too runny. Combine the remaining 1 teaspoon chamomile and 1 teaspoon cacao in a separate shallow dish. Pinch off ¼-teaspoon-sized pieces of the herb-honey mixture and roll into a ball between your palms. If the pills are sticking to your palms, coating your hands in a thin layer of coconut oil will solve the problem. Then roll each pill in the chamomile-cacao blend to coat.

Set your pills on parchment paper in a dehydrator on the lowest setting (to maintain the integrity of the honey do not dry above 95°F if possible) for 12 to 24 hours to dry completely. Alternatively, you can place them on a parchment paper–lined baking sheet in a breezy (not too breezy), but warm spot out of the sun to dry them completely, which could take up to 3 days. They will keep practically forever in a well-sealed jar in the refrigerator.

Headache Oxymel Herb Blend

This herb blend, as part of the oxymel trifecta with honey and apple cider vinegar, is my favorite remedy to release the tight, tense headaches that accompany caffeine withdrawal and dehydration. A dropperful of an oxymel with this herbal combination immediately goes to work on an achy head. **Makes 3 cups.**

½ cup dried chamomile flowers

¼ cup dried rosemary leaves

¼ cup dried thyme leaves and flowers

2 tablespoons dried lavender flowers

Use a quart jar and follow the directions on page 68 for preparing an oxymel. If you're planning to wean yourself off caffeine, be sure you start the process of making your oxymel at least 4 weeks before you make your commitment. Think of future you and set yourself up for success!

> **A small number of people are allergic to chamomile. You are more likely to be allergic to chamomile if you are already allergic to ragweed, daisies, or other members of the Asteraceae family. Try a small amount to start; if it brings you discomfort then this one's not for you.**

Soothing Eye Packs

Cucumber is cool and all, but chamomile works just as well on puffy eyes and dark circles. Plus, if you're traveling, it's a lot easier to stash a couple tea bags in your wallet, pocket, or carry-on than to keep a cucumber from getting crushed in transit and then wiping up slimy seeds. **Makes 2 eye packs.**

1 tablespoon dried chamomile flowers
or 2 chamomile tea bags

1 cup hot water

If you're at home, combine the chamomile flowers and the water in a bowl and let it steep for 7 to 10 minutes. Strain off the flowers and let the tea come to a comfortable temperature. Remember the skin around your eyes is more sensitive than the skin at your fingertips, so err on the side of cool. If you prefer cold, then pop the tea in the fridge to reach your desired temperature faster. Soak two cotton rounds or cuts from an old T-shirt in the tea and apply to closed eyes like you would two cucumber slices. If you're on the go you can substitute the tea and the cotton rounds for two chamomile tea bags. Hydrate them in warm or cool water, apply the bags to your eyes, and enjoy the eye packs in an airport, at a rest stop, or in your motel room.

Chickweed

Stellaria media

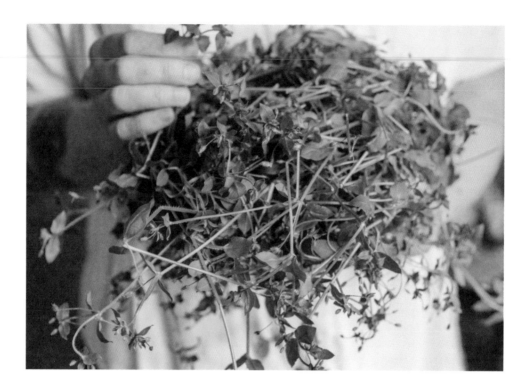

Reach for this when	You have itchy, irritated skin, there is diaper rash, a scab is healing, you have a cough, you're feeling achy and creaky in your joints, your insides are feeling parched, you're bored of eating spinach
Sensation	Cooling, moistening
Flavors	Sweet, salty, like corn silk or raw corn on the cob
Where it lives	Rich, moist, cultivated soil: front yards, untended areas of farms, neglected planters in a public park
Gather this	Anything above the ground, flowers and all, from fall to late spring
Super strengths	Demulcent, diuretic, alterative, nutritive, emollient, vulnerary

WHY I'M IN LOVE

Chickweed debuts each spring seemingly out of nowhere as one of the first gleams of green for our plant-starved eyes. I just love this plant's instinctual ability to protect. In storms, the small leaves fold up over the plant to protect the more vulnerable flowers and buds. And every night, it goes to "sleep" by folding over its buds, as well as partially closing its petals. Because it protects its own delicate structure so well, it can help us take care of ourselves too. Chickweed's botanical name *Stellaria media* roughly translates to "between the stars." Its long delicate stems crawl across the ground. In spring, the five white petals emerge, so deeply cut that they look like ten twinkling stars on a blanket of green. The common name "chickweed" comes from Europeans observing wild birds eating the plant, which is a good reminder that we're not the only ones who need it!

WHAT IT DOES BEST

Chickweed might be tiny, but it is certainly mighty. It is a nutritive powerhouse: rich in vitamins and minerals like potassium, magnesium, omega 3 and 6, vitamins A, B, C, calcium, chlorophyll, and iron. The combination of high mineral content and cooling actions make it an ideal remedy to a backed-up digestive system that may also experience hot expressions like ulcers. Chickweed is also high in a class of plant chemicals called saponins. Saponins are like soap; they get sudsy in water and even possess the soap-like ability to emulsify fat and water, neutralize toxins, dissolve fats (like how Dawn "cuts through grease"), and stimulate our mucus membranes. Saponins help our bodies do a better job absorbing the nutrient content of a plant. The saponins in chickweed mildly stimulate our mucus membranes, helping us trap and expel infection and can also encourage dry, hard coughs to be more productive.

Chickweed does powerful work inside our bodies but can also help heal and soothe almost anything that might be irritating the surface. It is a fast-acting healer of many wounds. It weakens, dissolves, and even consumes bacteria that cause infection and irritation on our skin. Applied as a poultice, oil, salve, or even added as a strong infusion to a bath, its soothing and cooling actions relieve eczema, psoriasis, bug bites, splinters and infected wounds, chicken pox, sores, blisters, diaper rash, and the general, forever mysterious itch. It is also an excellent lubricant for stiff, sore muscles and achy joints.

HOW IT GROWS

If a plant grows under the snow and no one is there to see it, can it be eaten? Yes! Chickweed is exactly that plant. It begins to grow in autumn, lives through the winter, makes seed like its life depends on it (it does) in spring, then dies when the weather gets warm around June. Chickweed likes the sun but prefers cool, shaded areas. It grows in every state of the continental United States. Chickweed itself is soft and flexible, which extends to our bodies. It is moved but not disturbed by strong winds, protects the most vulnerable parts of itself in rain, and even manages to be an effective groundcover by keeping soil from eroding. Like many of us, chickweed is fragile, but it doesn't fall apart. It protects itself and stays rooted to that which gives it life, but it is flexible enough to deal with whatever comes its way. It can be particularly of service when we feel ourselves holding tighter to refrains like "this is just how I am" or "I guess I'll never change."

TO RECAP

We are lucky to have a plant bearing so many gifts available to us in the doldrums of winter. This mineral-rich plant delivers optimum nutrition in winter and spring when green things are hard to come by and brings relief to a broad spectrum of symptoms that show up—particularly in the colder months. In March when the incessant blast of radiator heat feels inescapable, I turn to chickweed to soothe my dry, hot skin. The green tendrils slip easily into a simmering pot of soup or the bottom of a bowl as a nest for something warm. In the spring I am renewed by the soft, cold crunch it brings to the soups I've grown tired of eating, bringing vitality to my sleepy digestive system with its vitamin- and mineral-rich leaves and stems. Once you hold chickweed and experience its ability to maintain both vulnerability and strength, you will fall in love, be inspired by it, and feel excitement every time you notice its tiny stars keeping close to the earth.

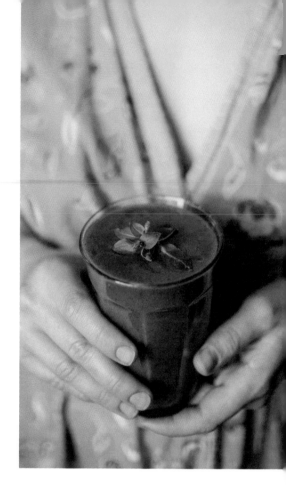

Weedy Smoothie

This is the drink I crave after the gym or a day spent in the sun. I know smoothies are a sugar fest, but if wild plants are involved it's fine by me. It's pretty easy to pluck chickweed from the earth without much effort: its shallow roots come up easily, much of the soil will fall off with a shake, and you can snip away the roots with ease. If you can't harvest your own, I'd guess that most farmers at your local greenmarket would be happy to sell you a generous bundle at a reasonable price like my favorite farmer does. **Makes 2 smoothies.**

½ cup orange juice

½ cup water

1 bunch fresh chickweed, rinsed and chopped (about 2 cups)

1 cup frozen pineapple chunks

Pour the orange juice and water into a blender, then add the chickweed and the pineapple. Cover and blend until smooth. Drink and enjoy this juicy, reviving smoothie.

Cooling Eye Balm

While the combination of chamomile and chickweed is great for the sensitive skin around our eyes, this formula works just as well as a lip balm or quick fix for irritated skin on any sensitive tissue (including the tiny bottoms of little ones). **Makes 10 lip balm tubes.**

SPECIAL EQUIPMENT: EMPTY LIP BALM TUBES OR TINS

1 tablespoon chickweed oil

1 tablespoon chamomile oil

1 tablespoon shea butter

1 tablespoon cocoa butter

2 tablespoons beeswax (either in pellet form or finely chopped from a larger piece)

Be sure to have made the chickweed and chamomile oil before beginning this process. Follow the directions for making an oil on page 80. I like to use olive oil for the chickweed oil and sesame oil for the chamomile oil. Additionally, I prefer using tubes for the eye balm so that I can easily apply under and around my eyes, on my lips, or around a chapped nose.

Combine the chickweed and chamomile oils with the shea butter, cocoa butter, and beeswax in a double boiler over low heat. Stir occasionally to distribute the beeswax evenly among the oils. Once the beeswax is completely dissolved, remove from the heat and pour immediately into tubes or short wide balm tins with screw tops. Do not store the balm in your glove compartment in case of melting.

Common Plantain

Plantago major

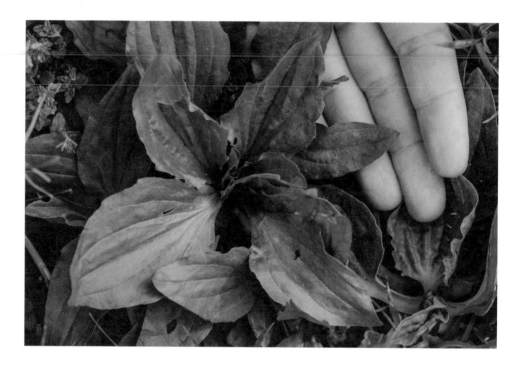

Reach for this when	Nursing an insect sting or bite, or minor wound, losing a lot of water because of sweating, diarrhea, or excessive urination, or when you need help opening up and flushing out your system
Sensation	Cooling, moistening
Flavors	Bitter, salty, earthy
Where it lives	Compacted soil, driveways, sidewalks, shaded fields
Gather this	Roots, leaves, flower spikes
Super strengths	Demulcent, diuretic, vulnerary, anti-inflammatory, antimicrobial, expectorant, nutritive, mildly astringent

WHY I'M IN LOVE

I could go on slathering calamine lotion on my bug bites but why would I when there's a plethora of plantain in the world? Plantain is your pal if you do literally anything outside that might get you minorly injured. Scrape your knee playing soccer? Plantain. Hornet sting you in your elbow crease? Plantain. SPF usage fail? Plantain, again. Make friends with plantain fast because you're going to need it when the sun is shining and the bugs are biting. It is the go-to remedy for the summer spectrum of minor catastrophes and pesky consequences of mother nature's gift of the warmth of the sun and our own failed environmental interventions. This is a nice way of saying that our world is not getting any colder. Make friends with the plants that will ease the pains of increasing humidity and heat. Plus, every time you choose plantain over a bottle of calamine lotion that's one less plastic bottle floating in the ocean.

WHAT IT DOES BEST

Plantain's greatest gift is its ability to suck out and keep in. Its nickname "snakeweed" comes from its famed skill of drawing snake venom from the body. I've not tried this for myself, nor have I seen it happen in real life, so don't take my word for it.

You don't have to wait for a snakebite (and I wouldn't advise you to), plantain can draw out irritation caused by bee, hornet, or wasp stings, mosquito and spider bites, as well as pus and infection from things like scrapped knees or pesky hangnails. The most amazing thing is that plantain leaves are an almost perfect bandage size. While yarrow is generally considered the plant for slowing minor bleeding, plantain is just as good and more likely to be around. If your body is sore from fluid loss, like if you've been crying or blowing your nose a lot, plantain can soothe the delicate skin around your eyes and your outer nose.

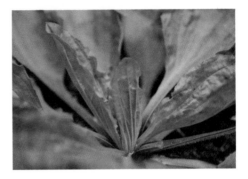

HOW IT GROWS

Common or broad-leaf plantain has 2- to 4-inch-long, wide leaves and parallel ribs that run the length of the leaf. Flower heads grow in compact spikes on long, straight leafless stalks. You can hardly walk in the world without stepping on it: it's in soccer fields, growing between the bricks of your patio, pushing up between sidewalk cracks, bursting from walls. The crappier and more compacted the soil the better.

TO RECAP

Most of the plants in this book are easy enough to find almost anywhere, but none are as prolific as plantain. It is among the most widely distributed medicinal plants in the entire world. Get plantaining people!

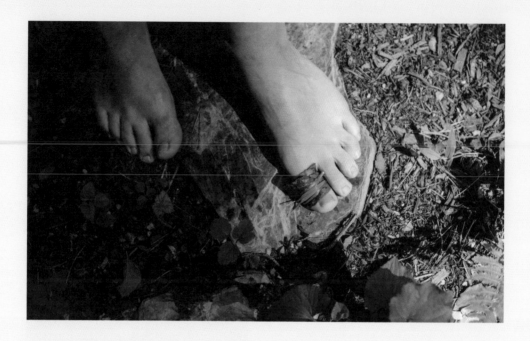

PLANTAIN BANDAGES AND SALVE

One wide, long plantain leaf is suitable for bites or stings on a finger, wrist, elbow crease, or toe. The fresh leaves, applied whole and bruised by scrunching them in your hand until the juices from the leaf are released, will almost instantly relieve the pain and inflammation of minor scrapes and insect bites or stings, but the longer you leave the bandage on the more healing it will confer. Step on a bee walking barefoot in the lawn? Wrap a plantain leaf around your toe and tie it off with a blade of grass and leave it on overnight. Need an extra punch? Chew up a few leaves and then slap the mush on the bite. Voila. Instant poultice and you don't even have to go inside.

Another remedy for itchy mosquito bites (as well as irritated hangnails or sensitive skin in general) is to make a plantain salve (see page 86). When gathering plantain take a dry measuring cup outside with you and locate a place that is free of pesticides and herbicides (steer clear of power lines, railroads, and downhill where runoff of water accumulates). Fill the cup with broad- or narrow-leaf plantain. If you don't feel confident you can locate safe plantain then you can purchase dried from a local medicinal farm or just regular farm (as we've already established plantain grows everywhere).

Digestive Repair Tea

If we put bandages on the outside of our bodies, why can't we do the same for our insides? Plantain can help our gut to heal in the same way it does our skin after a bug bite or sting. Digestive upset is pretty common: it doesn't take a lot to push our tummies toward rebellion. This infusion can help calm symptoms that result from inflamed and irritated gut upset and disease.
Makes 3 cups.

3 cups water

2 teaspoons dried plantain leaf

2 teaspoons dried marshmallow root

1 teaspoon dried rose petals

1 teaspoon dried chamomile flowers

1 teaspoon dried cinnamon chips

1 teaspoon dried fennel seed

1 teaspoon dried mint leaves

Boil the water, turn off the heat, and let it sit while you combine the herbs in a quart jar. Cover the herbs with the slightly cooled water, cap, and put in the refrigerator overnight. Sip over ice during the day to ease and strengthen your stomach.

Dandelion

Taraxacum officinale

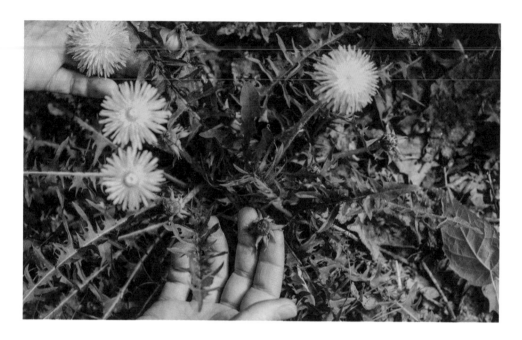

Reach for this when	You are coming off a sugar bender, it's spring and time to eat green things again, you need some cheering up in the dead of winter
Sensation	Cooling, drying
Flavors	Flowers: sweet Leaves: bitter, earthy Roots: bitter, salty
Where it lives	Disturbed earth, city parks, suburban lawns, edge of forest bordering trails, wild meadows, cracks in sidewalks, walls
Gather this	Flowers: spring and summer Leaves: spring (least bitter) through fall (most bitter) Roots: fall
Super strengths	Tonic, diuretic, alterative, antirheumatic, bitter, cholagogue, hepatic, exhilarant, mild laxative, nutritive

WHY I'M IN LOVE

I can't consider my childhood without seeing dandelions. They were everywhere and I was obsessed with digging them up. Fortunately, I was a terrible digger, unable to get the tricky taproot completely free from the soil. But I loved the fight that the dandelion put up, the long spindly, broken root that emerged, and the assurance that in a few weeks there would be more. Every summer I collect its sunny flowers and tincture them in vodka or preserve them in honey. When winter arrives and inevitably gets tough—I miss the sun, I miss the contact with people, I retreat inside myself—I look on my herb shelves for my jar of liquid sunshine. I take a half dropperful and am instantly exhilarated. While dandelion leaves and roots relieve chronic stagnation in the liver, dandelion flowers can relieve a stagnant, depressed spirit. I guess now is an appropriate time to confess that dandelion is my favorite plant. I love it for being scrappy, fierce, life giving, and cheery.

WHAT IT DOES BEST

The modern scientific name for dandelion is the first clue of dandelion's healing power. The genus name comes from the Greek *taraxos*, meaning a disorder, and *akos*, meaning a remedy. Whenever you see *officinale* following the genus name you know that this plant is kind of a big deal. If you were to travel back in time you would likely find this plant in ancient pharmacies or the *officina*. For thousands of years people relied on these plants and they've been used in the practice of medicine ever since. Dandelion basically means the official remedy for any disorder.

Working from the ground up, dandelion roots are the source of its strength. If you are experiencing sluggish digestion, go for a bitter root like dandelion. You can think of it this way: dandelion root kicks the digestive system into high gear like coffee does but without the stimulant of caffeine. Why should you care? Because if your digestive system is slow then everything else suffers.

Dandelion root also improves bile production in the liver, which means that you can digest fats and eliminate toxins from your body with way more ease. Isn't that a relief? Speaking of relief, dandelion root is also a mild laxative. Ahem, the coffee correlation. Dandelion is high in mineral content and inulin, a type of fiber, which is an excellent prebiotic as well.

It may not come as a surprise that just as we are gearing up for a summer of salads and fresh fruit, the bitter leaves of dandelion appear. It's like nature knows our digestive systems have been slow all winter. Dandelion is here to wake us up from our diet of sleepy soups made from thick roots and bones (and beer!). Dandelion is a tonic, and during the spring we can eat it and take it as medicine every day. That's the point of a tonic—take it every day, and little by little, we improve. It is the ultimate preventative medicine. It's high in potassium too!

HOW IT GROWS

From the first flush of blooms in early spring, dandelion season lasts until snow covers the ground. From each dandelion root sprouts a rosette of leaves, so long as there are green leaves, they are edible. They do get progressively more bitter throughout the season so you may want to begin with tender spring leaves. From the leaves of each plant sprouts a single stem supporting a single flower. One dandelion plant can produce more than 2,000 seeds, though some reports say it is as much as 20,000. Dandelion reproduces without pollination—the seeds ride the wind and go places. This determined spirit is perhaps my favorite of dandelion's qualities.

Blooms appear throughout the spring, summer, and early fall. Dandelion is in the daisy family, Asteraceae, which also happens to be the largest flowering plant family. Its name indicates that the flower heads are composites of individual flowers. How cool is that? The head of a dandelion flower is actually lots and lots of individual flowers.

Dandelion grows almost anywhere: wild in fields, lining trails, in suburban yards, breaking through cracks of city sidewalks, and in the disturbed earth of forgotten city construction sites. Its constant presence is a reminder of its persistence to live as long as it can under any condition.

TO RECAP

Dandelion stimulates digestion without the caffeine jitters, is full of good things for the tiny guys populating our gut, and offers dynamic mineral-rich nutrition. What does this mean for everything outside our digestive systems? Good digestion and regular liver cleansing mean better health overall. For one thing, having the support of dandelion means we get a break from all of the metabolic processing our bodies do all the time. With dandelion lightening the load, the liver is better able to support the cleaning and thinning of the blood, which means the overall quality of our blood is improved. Liver clearance, clean blood, and high mineral content also means inflammation in our bodies goes down. Our skin also looks better. Everything in and on our bodies is connected, and in order to see healthful change we need to find ways to support the organs at the root of our illnesses, however large or small, physical or spiritual.

Winter Rescue Tincture

I make this tincture in early summer when I feel as alive with possibility as the earth. Come winter time, I am in serious need of some sunshine. A dropperful throughout the day of this simple medicine moves me out of my dreary disposition and gears me up for welcoming spring and all of its renewal. **Makes about 2 cups.**

1½ cups dandelion flower blossoms (I use the entire top)

1 cup honey

1 cup brandy

Put the flowers in a glass pint jar. Dissolve the honey in the brandy by stirring or whisking vigorously together. Pour the brandy and honey over the flowers, label, and store in a cool, dark place for 6 weeks. Bottle your tincture, but don't hide it away so well that you forget about it by winter!

Hillary's Morning Brew

My friend Hillary made a variation of this caffeine-free coffee substitute when I was visiting her in Oakland. Her apartment is surrounded by persimmon, fig, and lemon trees. This drink is as gently coaxing as a bright fall morning in the East Bay. **Makes 1 drink.**

1 cup milk of choice

1 teaspoon chopped roasted dandelion root

1 teaspoon chopped roasted chicory root

Pinch of ground clove

Spoonful of honey

Add the milk to a small saucepan and warm over medium heat until tiny bubbles gather around the edge of the pan. When steam rises from the pan, add the dandelion root, chicory root, and ground clove. Let it steep for 6 minutes, then re-warm and whisk vigorously to froth the milk. Put your spoonful of honey in a mug and pour the hot liquid through a sieve or cheesecloth into the mug to melt the honey into the drink.

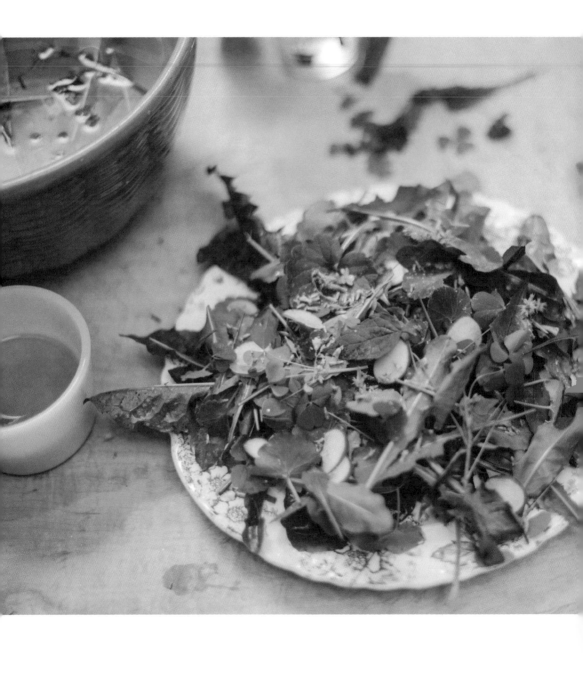

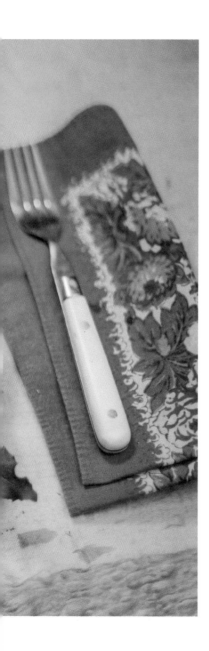

Yard Salad

Ultra-nutritious dandelion is jam packed with vitamins A, E, K, B6, B2, B1, and C. That's more than spinach *or* broccoli! Its leaves are bitter, but you can easily temper the young spring growth with other ingredients. I like to fill a big salad bowl with dandelion leaves, wood sorrel, plantain leaves, and garden herbs. You can add toasted seeds or nuts, dried fruit, shaved cheese, and some protein if you really want to make a meal out of it! **Serves 4.**

6 cups dandelion leaves and other foraged or purchased greens and herbs

2 tablespoons lemon juice, from half a juicy lemon or a whole not-so-juicy lemon

½ teaspoon sea salt

1 teaspoon local, raw honey

2 teaspoons Dijon mustard

½ teaspoon black pepper

¼ cup plus 1 tablespoon olive oil

Wash the leaves and greens and place in a large bowl. Combine the lemon juice with the salt and honey in a small bowl, stir to dissolve the honey and salt. Next add the mustard and black pepper and slowly drizzle the olive oil in as you whisk to emulsify the dressing. Toss your salad with the dressing and serve with crusty bread, grilled meat, or soup!

Eastern White Pine

Pinus strobus

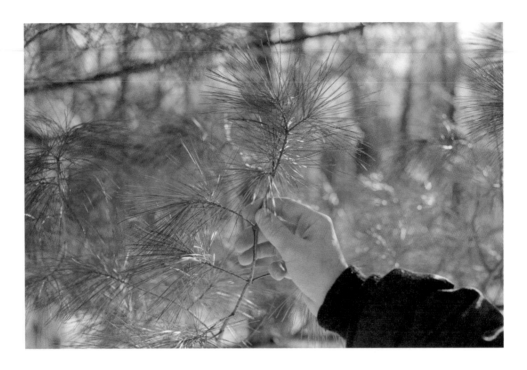

Reach for this when	You need to get things moving or bring things together, you're looking for a feeling of restorative peace
Sensation	Warming, sticky, drying
Flavors	Pungent
Where it lives	From the mountains to the sea, in temperate parts of eastern North America, in urban parks, forests, and yards
Gather this	Needles, resin
Super strengths	Anti-inflammatory, analgesic, anticatarrhal, nutritive, carminative, diuretic, antimicrobial, astringent

WHY I'M IN LOVE

When I drive from the city into the hills of the Catskills, the scent of pine trees pours through my windows and immediately calms my busy body and mind. I experience the same feeling when wandering into a part of a city park where only pines grow, standing atop the dried needles from winters before, closing my eyes and being overcome with the soothing aroma of the trees. After breathing deep for a few minutes, I feel an abiding calm and I also feel more awake. As a native conifer, the Eastern white pine holds a significant space in the history of peace for the indigenous people of the Haudenosaunee Confederacy or People of the Longhouse. The Great White Pine stands at the center of their story as the Tree of Peace that united five nations: Mohawks, Oneidas, Onondagas, Cayugas, and Senecas. Had it not been for indigenous knowledge of viable winter food from native flora like pine, most colonists would have likely died over the winter from diseases like scurvy. Standing at the base of a giant pine or in the company of young trees beginning their lives is to experience an overwhelming sense of peace and possibility. The tree also offers a constant reminder that we are on indigenous land and that we must take responsibility and remediate the suffering caused by the people they helped keep alive.

WHAT IT DOES BEST

The resin the tree produces as part of its own immune system has a bringing-together-type healing effect. When a tree sustains an injury, like a limb falling off or being cut into, it rushes sap to the area and releases resin as a kind of scab. The resin of soft pines such as the Eastern white pine is relatively runny compared to other pines, but as it dries it gets firmer to patch the wound. If you harvest resin from an open wound on the tree, you'll lose your own limbs as punishment. That's not true, but it should be because the tree needs the resin to properly heal and protect itself against infection. While it's very generous of the tree to produce the resin, it's not actually intended for you. You may collect the fresh resin that drips onto parts of the tree below the wound or the resin that falls to the ground. The dried resin resembles bird poop but is easily distinguishable from the real thing.

If you have a splinter, a slightly inflamed wound, or ingrown hair, applying a thin paste of fresh resin can expedite the healing process by gently stimulating the local immune response to push the splinter (or whatever) up and out and bring your wound back together. The resin is strongly antimicrobial, and when applied topically, it cleans while comfortably relieving your skin of the obstruction. I've even seen it work on a tiny shard of glass lodged in a heel.

HOW IT GROWS

You can easily identify Eastern white pine by its clusters of five long needles, a leaf adaptation by evergreen trees to endure cold, dry winters. The needles meet at a single point and aren't completely smooth when you roll them between your thumb and forefinger. Every needle has a white stripe going up one side, hence "white pine." Practice restraint when harvesting needles, branches, and resin. If you can, and you probably can, only harvest needles from branches and twigs that fall to the ground after a rain or snowstorm.

TO RECAP

As one of few viable wild food sources in the wintertime to animals, and at one time humans, white pine offers numerous remedies. Its needles are high in vitamin C making it a super preventer of cold and flu when taken internally as an infusion. Pine can help relieve symptoms associated with coughs and bronchitis by gently stimulating the lungs and relaxing our airways to help move out stuck phlegm. Try an infusion or steam bath of the needles or just suck on some of the dried resin! A delightful way to ease the aches and creaks of a cold, dry winter body is to bathe in a white pine infusion. Adding a quart to your tub is a trifecta: it soothes joints and muscles, relaxes the airways, and prepares the body and mind for deep, restorative, peaceful rest.

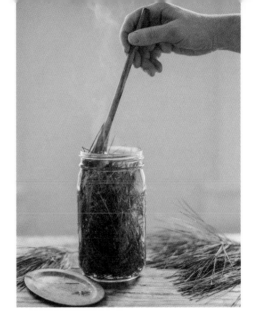

Evergreen Syrup

A syrup of pine needles is a delightful remedy for a cough, high in vitamin C, and beneficial for our lungs. A spoonful of this syrup reminds us that vibrant health is possible even if it's hard to find during the winter season. **Makes 2½ cups.**

1 cup cut and sifted white pine needles

1 cup honey or other sweetener

2 tablespoons brandy

Fill a glass quart jar with the white pine needles, cover with hot water up to where the neck of the bottle begins, cap, and let sit at room temperature for 8 to 12 hours. Strain off and compost the needles, and pour the liquid into a measuring cup. Note the amount of liquid before transferring to a saucepan. Bring the infusion to just below a simmer on low heat and reduce to 1½ cups. Stir in the honey and brandy. Refrigerated between uses, this syrup will last 6 months.

Winter Soup Seasoning

Many evergreens make great seasoning. The flavor of white pine is mild and happens to be one of my favorites; I like it on stewed white beans or in chicken soup. Spruce needles are even stronger and can be used in place of rosemary (great for heavier stews of red meats!). **Makes about ⅓ cup.**

SPECIAL EQUIPMENT: DEHYDRATOR

6 small branches (about ¼-inch thick) of white pine needles

Prepare your needles by plucking them in groups of five from the branch and rinsing them in cool water. Use a dehydrator or the lowest setting on your oven to dry them until they snap when bent. The dehydrator method may take about 10 hours at 120°F. In the oven, I like to dry them at around 180°F for half an hour then turn it off and let them sit for a half hour more. Once dry, grind them in a blender or coffee grinder. Use as you would any seasoning powder.

Forest Vinegar

This is a balsamic-type vinegar that can be used on salads and vegetables. **Makes 1½ cups.**

1 cup pine needles, finely chopped

1 cup apple cider vinegar

Add the pine needles to a glass pint jar and cover with the vinegar, making sure all the needles are completely covered by 1 inch of vinegar. Place wax paper or plastic wrap over the top of the jar, screw on the lid tightly, and put in a cool dark place. Leave for at least 2 weeks—1 month is better—before straining into a pretty bottle with a non-reactive cover. Use like you would any balsamic vinegar. It's mildly sweet but packed with vitamin C, which is something our bodies crave until Florida citrus hits the shelves sometime midwinter.

Garlic

Allium sativum

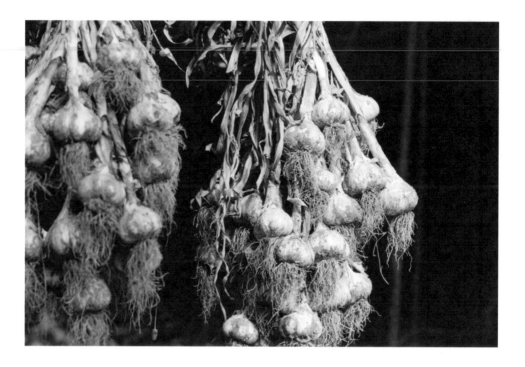

Reach for this when	Almost any time you are preparing food, when you feel a cold coming on, for heart and cardiovascular health in general
Sensation	Warming
Flavors	Sweet, bitter
Where it lives	Rich, moist soil, such as in farmers' fields
Gather this	The bulb
Super strengths	Rubefacient, tonic, antiseptic, antimicrobial, antispasmodic, carminative, diaphoretic, expectorant, stimulant, diuretic, nutritive, cardiotonic, antifungal

WHY I'M IN LOVE

Garlic is probably most famous for warding off vampires. It's been suggested that this folklore originated with Europeans who witnessed the ravaging of diseases like rabies, tuberculosis, or plague. Without a lot of available information in the form of precise medical diagnoses, they compensated with supernatural explanations. The gaunt bodies of the infirmed or decomposing oozed blood and exhibited receding gums and long nails. In fact the word *nosferatu*, which was used in Bram Stoker's *Dracula* originates in the Greek word *nosophorus* meaning "plague carrier." Physicians, healers, clergy, sailors, soldiers, and thieves relied on garlic in treating all of the aforementioned diseases. Garlic, it just so happens, is a broad-spectrum antimicrobial, among other strengths, so while I'm not worried about vampires, there's plenty of disease to throw cloves at.

WHAT IT DOES BEST

Garlic is a protective herb against many vampires that masquerade as modern disease. When eaten often and regularly, garlic encourages the body's natural defense against bacteria, viruses, and fungal infection. It shortens the duration of illness, like the common cold for example, by stimulating the immune system, thinning mucus, and helping the body produce an effective fever. Garlic also eases the discomfort of illness. Its gently warming and moistening actions are well-suited to situations that are stiff, stuck, or clogged. Garlic is great for chronic conditions: Same old ear infection coming back? Get the same cough around the end of December year after year? Lost your appetite? Can't get rid of it? Reach for a well-known remedy the world over: garlic.

Popularly regarded as a panacea since antiquity, garlic may actually be worthy of the title. Lots of plants are peddled as panaceas, mostly by people who want to make money, but not all plants are for all situations, they're not even for all people! Garlic is not for everyone either: some people may experience discomfort after consuming or applying garlic.

A simple way to allay the likelihood of illness is to eat more plants that are good for us—like highly nutritive garlic—because the spread of and suffering from disease is partially due to poor nutrition. Garlic is also healing to our cardiovascular system; it can lower blood pressure by relaxing the smooth muscle cells of our vascular system. We knew way back when that garlic could ward off disease and even help us fight it once our bodies succumbed to it. We now know why. We also know that we're more likely to reap its benefits if we ingest it regularly and consistently—wearing it as a necklace won't cut it.

HOW IT GROWS

The garlic we eat is a bulb that belongs to the onion family. Native to the Mediterranean, it is planted in the fall in rich soil in full sun. Some varieties produce flower-bearing scapes, which you can find in abundance at farmers markets in the summer. Many of us purchase garlic that has been cured (tied together and hung in a cool dark place for 3 weeks to form the characteristic papery skin enclosing the individual cloves).

TO RECAP

Garlic is an easy way to get good medicine through the food we eat; it doesn't ask us to change a whole lot about how we live our lives, only that it be included. We can enjoy it raw or cooked. But always smash, bruise, or cut garlic before consuming it to release the allicin that's responsible for a lot of the good work garlic does in your body.

Fermented Garlic Honey

I'm a big believer in having things around that are good for me and ready to go, like this fermented garlic honey. With a few simple ingredients and a little bit of time, you'll be equipped to tackle any cold or sore throat that creeps your way. **Makes about 1 cup.**

SPECIAL EQUIPMENT: PH TESTING STRIPS (AVAILABLE AT MANY DRUGSTORES)

1 medium-large head garlic, peeled and smashed (about ½ cup)

1 cup honey

Apple cider vinegar (optional)

Put the garlic in a wide-mouth glass pint jar and add the honey (it should completely cover the garlic cloves but be sure to leave 1½ inches between the honey-garlic mixture and the lid). Place the lid on the jar loosely, then tuck into a dark place. Every few days burp the jar (unscrewing the lid to release the gas) and flip it over. After 3 days or so bubbles should start to form. Over time the honey will get increasingly liquidy. If you're worried about botulism you can test with litmus pH strips to make sure the preparation is under 4.6 pH. If it's creeping up, add a splash of apple cider vinegar to bring it back down. Ferment for at least 1 week, after which point you'll have a sweet garlicky syrup and tasty little garlic morsels. Take a clove with a spoonful of honey when you feel a cold coming on.

Everyday Medicinal Broth

Homemade broth should be in every home healers tool kit. Growing up, it was a true cure-all in my house: my mum used broth to heal and ease a wide variety of illnesses from real flus to made-up ones. Straight up chicken broth is delicious, but given the opportunity to pump it up, why wouldn't you? I especially love a garlicky broth in the late days of winter as our bodies get ready for spring. Making broth medicinal doesn't require an exotic escapade, just head to your grocery store for all your medicine-making needs! **Makes about 6 cups.**

1 organic chicken carcass (see sidebar)

2 tablespoons apple cider vinegar

1 onion, quartered, skin on

1 bunch thyme

1 bunch rosemary

2 sheets kombu

1 tablespoon black peppercorns

3 heads garlic

Put the chicken carcass, apple cider vinegar, and onion in a large stockpot or slow cooker and cover with water. Set the lid, turn the heat to low, and simmer for 8 to 12 hours. Add the thyme, rosemary, kombu, pepper-corns, and garlic. Cover and let the broth continue to simmer for an hour longer and then turn off the heat. When the stock has cooled a bit, strain the liquid into a bowl and set up an ice bath to quickly and safely cool the broth. Store in airtight containers in the fridge and use within 4 to 5 days. If you don't think you can get through the broth within 5 days, then you can freeze it in ice cube trays or muffin tins and then store the cubes or disks in reusable storage containers.

Though I do recommend you buy organic whenever you are able, sometimes it might be out of your budget or simply not available. The chicken in this recipe is one case where I really must insist on organic only because a long, low extraction from bones means any chemicals and toxins administered to the animal throughout its life is then stored in the bones and the marrow and will leach into your broth. I'm not interested in drinking any bad stuff and I wouldn't want anyone else to ingest it either.

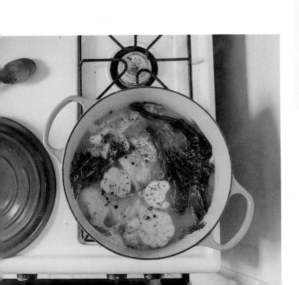

Ginger

Zingiber officinale

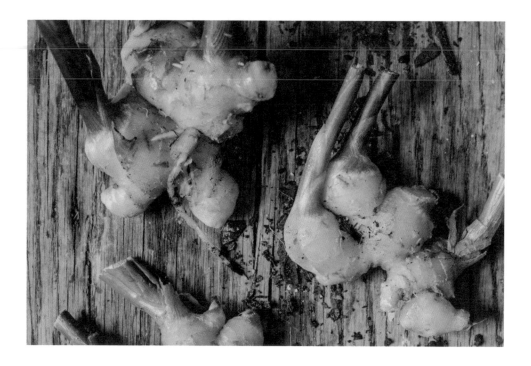

Reach for this when	You need to soothe a nauseated stomach, get your blood moving from your center to your periphery, kick a cold to the curb
Sensation	Hot, dry
Flavors	Spicy, pungent, floral, and fruity
Where it lives	Hot, humid environments, tropical regions, container gardens, rich and moist soil
Gather this	Ginger is a rhizome (an underground stem); it's never out of season in the grocery store
Super strengths	Diaphoretic, stimulant, emmenagogue, antispasmodic, anti-microbial, anti-inflammatory, carminative

WHY I'M IN LOVE

When I was in college, my friends and I would have juice parties (we were nerds with glowing skin!). When everyone else went to the liquor store, we'd go to the natural food store to buy up the produce section. We started with tasty combinations before moving on to single plant shots. I will never forget my first shot of ginger—my first thought of "this is no big deal, I feel warm" was quickly followed by the sensation of breathing fire. The heat resonated from my stomach up through my esophagus and out my salivating mouth. With warmth penetrating every tissue of my body, a wave of heat built and moved throughout to expel whatever was cold and tense. You should definitely try it.

WHAT IT DOES BEST

Ginger is not so different from a fire that burns logs but also warms everything around it. A bunch of ginger in your body is like stoking a fire in your core that moves out to warm us from head to toe. As movement is stimulated and blood moves through our muscle tissues, they relax, easing any pain associated with tension and making pathways for our blood to move all the way to our skin. Ginger can help facilitate a productive fever by encouraging the skin to open so that the heat it generates has an exit point. After we heal, ginger leaves our skin looking radiant and bright.

Ginger is particularly helpful for pain that feels stuck. If what you experience can be described with words like tense, heavy, cold, slow, constrictive, clamped, cramped, gripping, congested, or hard, then consider working with ginger. The first place we are likely to feel these sensations is in our digestive system, which is made up of very active organs, so when they slow down and get stuck that can mean upset elsewhere. As soon as we put ginger on our tongues our salivary glands signal the body to get the digestive process going. Ginger relieves stagnation by moving blood to places that experience tension, helping them to relax. While this action initiates in our digestive system, we might experience it in our pelvis to relieve a stagnant menstrual cycle or in our heads to ease a tight headache. When applied topically to areas that feel inflamed or stiff and cold, ginger will call blood to flood the area. By bringing blood to the site of pain ginger relaxes the muscles around our arteries making it easy for our blood to move from our core to the more distant parts of ourselves like pinky toes reminding us that we are all one body.

HOW IT GROWS

Ginger grows naturally in tropical locations. While it prefers heat and humidity, ginger is container friendly: it requires a shady home in the corner of a summer garden, roof, or patio and to be brought indoors in the cooler months. While the part of the ginger plant that we most commonly consume is referred to as a root, this is actually a misnomer. Ginger is a rhizome or an underground stem with sprouting stems that grow up and roots that grow down and are more fibrous.

TO RECAP

All the chemical elements that come together to make up ginger activate the many organs, systems, and pathways in our body that help us to feel relaxed and comfortable. Ginger improves our digestive process, relieves headaches, regulates menses, and even modulates our body temperature. In the process, it reminds us that our bodies, which are also comprised of many elements, can work together toward balance and comfort. Ginger is the friend you need when you, or parts of you, have been sitting around too long: it will come to your house, bust down the door, and get you moving.

Fire Cider

Fire cider is a well-known and well-loved home remedy that is simple to prepare and delicious to drink. I like to take shots of it when I have to head out early on my bike in the winter or when I feel an illness coming on. Its super delicious as a zippy addition to a mugful of warm bone broth. **Makes 3 cups.**

¾ cup packed grated ginger
(use large-hole grater)

½ cup packed grated horseradish
(use large-hole grater)

¾ cup chopped onion

¼ cup chopped garlic

Zest of 1 lemon

2 tablespoons grated turmeric

1 tablespoon chopped rosemary

¼ teaspoon powdered cayenne

2 cups apple cider vinegar

¼ cup honey

Combine all the ingredients except the apple cider vinegar and honey in a glass quart jar. Pour the vinegar over the mixture and cap with a plastic lid or a couple layers of plastic wrap underneath a metal one. Shake thoroughly and label with the date. Place in a cool, dark place for 4 to 6 weeks, but remember to shake the jar every few days. (If you think you'll forget about it, then leave it on your counter out of direct sunlight.) After 4 to 6 weeks strain the liquid off the solids; use a cheesecloth to twist and turn to squeeze every last drop of cider from the plants. Stir in the honey. Bottle the cider vinegar and keep it in your fridge for 6 months.

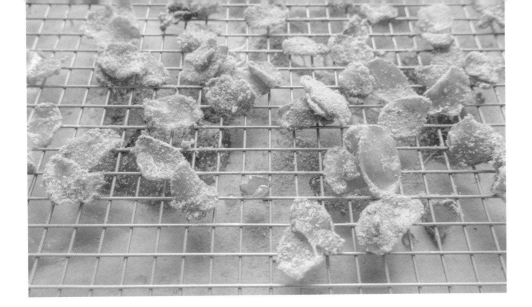

Maple Candied Ginger

Ginger is probably most famous for soothing nausea from sea sickness to looking at your phone while in a cab. It is also a part of my mother's remedy for the stomach flu: ginger ale and saltine crackers. This is one of ginger's special powers: its ability to calm nausea from *any* source. Ginger swoops in to offer swift relief whether our nausea begins on land or at sea, during pregnancy, or from illness. Note that fresh ginger in the late summer or early fall will be less spicy and pungent than ginger from the grocery store.

Makes 2 cups.

SPECIAL EQUIPMENT: CANDY THERMOMETER

½ pound ginger

½ cup maple syrup

1 teaspoon coconut oil or other vegetable oil

¼ cup maple sugar

If you want, peel the ginger by using the side of a small spoon to scrape the outer layer off. Slice the ginger as thin as possible, add to a small saucepan, and cover with the maple syrup. Set over medium heat and bring to a simmer, about 5 minutes. In the meantime, set up a baking sheet lined with parchment paper. Place a cooling rack on top of the parchment and brush the rack with the coconut oil. When the mixture has come to a simmer, reduce heat to medium low and simmer for 25 minutes, stirring often. In the last 5 minutes begin to take the temperature, tipping the saucepan so the syrupy ginger falls to one side and you can get a good read. When the thermometer reads 250°F, pull it off the heat and let it sit for ½ hour. Strain and reserve the syrup for waffles, pancakes, or oatmeal. Then scatter the candied ginger onto the cooling rack, wait 3 minutes, then work quickly to separate the sticky slices. Dust with the maple sugar and allow to dry. The candy will keep for 3 months in the refrigerator. It's not only a fantastic remedy for motion sickness but also good for those of us without fireplaces in winter.

Hawthorn

Crataegus spp.

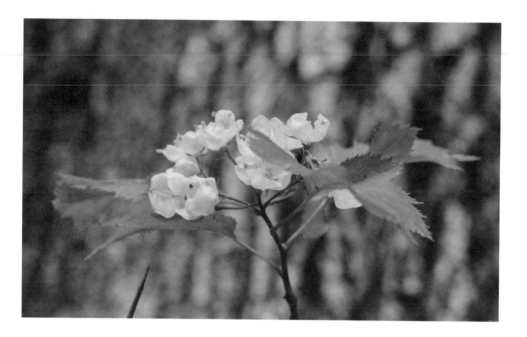

Reach for this when	Prolonged physical or emotional stress has you feeling over excited and weak, you've been chowing on Cheetos lately, you've got some big things to confront or let go
Sensation	Cool, dry, tonifying
Flavors	Berries: sweet, some describe as overripe apples Flowers: nutty, slightly astringent
Where it lives	Prefers the sun, popular in cities because they're tolerant of pollution, in parks growing like trees or shrubs, in the liminal space between country and town, near moist soil (likely to find a small creek nearby)
Gather this	Leaves, berries
Super strengths	Exhilarant, relaxant, diuretic, astringent, nervine, stomachic, antioxidant, cardiotonic

WHY I'M IN LOVE

At certain times of year, I have to really look for hawthorn. I have to think about it, want to find it, and then pay attention when I'm out in the world scanning the landscape. I know of one tree in Prospect Park near where I live, but all the other times I've happened upon it I've exclaimed out loud, "But *is* it?" Not because I'm unsure of identifying it, but I just don't see it that often. I duck under the sprawling, bushy branches examining the flowers and looking for the telltale thorns. Hawthorns thorns, which are botanically speaking true thorns, are long and widely spaced, making it an ideal habitat for nesting—or resting—birds. It's delightful under the canopy of a hawthorn: cool, guarded, removed ever so slightly from the carrying-on just beyond its thorny bows. Hawthorn is famous for being protective both in its medicine and in its nature. It is an ideal medicine, physically and emotionally, for navigating situations that require a lot of attention: big shifts, a chronic condition, or embarking on a big transition are no match for hawthorn.

WHAT IT DOES BEST

Hawthorn is maybe best known as a strengthening and uplifting heart medicine. Though hawthorn is gentle and safe, it is also powerful and nourishing to the cardiovascular system. It brings balance through protection by increasing the strength of the heart muscle, helping the right amount of blood get to the heart so it has enough oxygen to do its work, and lowering blood pressure. In these ways hawthorn at once prevents and mitigates damage to the organs and functions of our cardiovascular system. If you already have low blood pressure, consult a professional before beginning a course of therapy that includes hawthorn.

As humans we aim to avoid oxidative stress: our bodies prefer to counteract the damaging effects of free radicals by neutralizing them with antioxidants. Free radicals bounce around our bodies stealing electrons from other atoms in our cells and tissues. They end up damaging cells, proteins, and even our DNA, which can contribute to type 2 diabetes, autoimmune disease, and cardiovascular disease. Free radicals come from lifestyle choices like smoking, not getting enough sleep, sitting around all day, environmental toxins like air pollution and plastics, chronic stress and anxiety, industrial vegetable oils, plus not getting enough antioxidants in our diet. Some of these things are hard for us to change, but its relatively easy to identify fruits and vegetables high in antioxidants: they're colorful! Hawthorn berries are an excellent source of antioxidants. They can clear out free radicals, protect our arterial walls from injury, and reduce oxidative damage to capillary walls.

HOW IT GROWS

Hawthorn is a slow grower with many trees living to be over 100 years old! Like other members of the rose family, its flowers have five petals. Hawthorn blooms around May, which is why it is popularly known as May Tree. The blooms often have an off-putting scent to some. The leaves tend to vary, even within the same species, though they are generally lobed. The thorns are often at least an inch long, widely spaced, and sharp. The fruit ripens in the fall and may be collected through the end of October. The berries range from bright to deep, dark red and are slightly waxy.

TO RECAP

Hawthorn is a great ally for warding off or reducing the harmful effects of some pretty big threats. It is a safe plant that protects our heart, delivers antioxidants, and supports the function of our cardiovascular system. Emotionally, it provides the space to reflect on and respond to big life events whether you're in the midst of a crisis or taking the opportunity to anticipate and move through a particularly challenging moment.

Hawthorn Cordial

This tasty fall cordial supports and strengthens the heart as well as the digestive system as it works to nourish and support the rest of the body. Enjoy the cordial with friends and family; it is delightful with sparkling water as a pre-dinner drink for those of us who prefer a cocktail with a little less punch and a little more medicine. **Makes about 2 cups.**

1 medium apple, peeled and roughly chopped into 1-inch pieces

1 cup dried hawthorn berries

One 3-inch cinnamon stick

One 1-inch-thick peel from a lemon

Pinch of ground cardamom

1½ cups brandy

½ cup honey

Put the apple chunks, hawthorn berries, cinnamon sticks, lemon peel and cardamom in a glass pint jar. Combine the brandy and honey in a liquid measure and then pour over the mixture in the jar. Shake thoroughly and label with the date. Place in a cool dark place for 4 weeks, remembering to shake the jar daily. After 4 weeks, strain off the solids and compost the plant material. This is a delicious cordial to have after dinner with dessert to aid digestion and stabilize your blood sugar, especially in cooler fall and winter months.

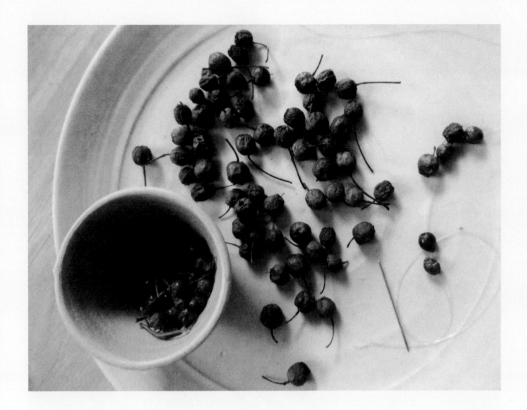

HAWTHORN NECKLACE

It's rare that you can make jewelry out of flowers and leaves, unless you're particularly skilled. Berries are another story! I like to make a necklace of rose hips and hawthorn berries so that I have their energies close to my heart, a place where their medicine and emotional protection are best felt. To start, gather enough hawthorn berries to string on a necklace. You may want to include rose hips or other beads, berries, or stones that resonate with you. Get wild! Using a tapestry needle and fishing line string the berries while they're still fresh. Be sure to snuggle them up because as they dry they'll shrink. Affix a fastener on either end and wear your necklace on days when you need a little extra encouragement: traversing the TSA, a first date, or visiting a loved one in the hospital.

Lemon Balm

Melissa officinalis

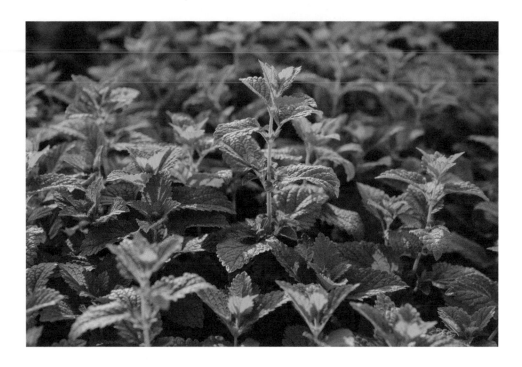

Reach for this when	You're feeling anxious and can't sleep, having a herpes outbreak, mild restless tension, stomach upset, or headache
Sensation	Cooling, drying
Flavors	Aromatic, sour
Where it lives	Wastelands, bordering houses and fences breaking at the sidewalk, in the alleyways behind houses, bordering walking paths
Gather this	Leaves, flowers
Super strengths	Nervine, relaxant, antiviral, antispasmodic, diaphoretic, sedative, anodyne

WHY I'M IN LOVE

If I could build a house from any plant, it would surely be lemon balm. My home is a place where I am safe and where I establish practices and routines that keep me healthy and nurtured by relationships with friends, family, and pets. The effects of lemon balm encourage a state of being that facilitates all of those things: it's uplifting, restorative, and calming. Moving through life with ease and calm is easier said than done, but lemon balm can be just the ally when trying to cultivate a less hectic life, especially at home.

WHAT IT DOES BEST

Lemon balm is a gentle, but effective nervine. It calms anxiety, soothes nervous tension, relieves headaches and stomachaches, and eases insomnia. I find it particularly helpful when any of these situations are precipitated by or aggravated due to exhaustion: the toddler who wants to play in the middle of the night (read: my nephew), the parents who have to go to work after a sleepless night (my sister and her husband), a childless adult burning the midnight oil to write her book before going back to her full-time job the next day (doesn't sound like anyone I know). Lemon balm quiets the restlessness that comes along with being overtired. Sleep is in many ways our first line of defense and a cornerstone of foundational health combined with eating healthfully, exercising, and drinking enough water. But sleep is often the first thing to suffer whenever life gets demanding and without adequate sleep we're left more vulnerable

to making unhealthy choices. We are more likely to reach for something sugary and processed to give us a superficial energy boost just to get through the day. The combination of sleepless nights and junk food makes our bodies prime playgrounds for viruses like colds and flus.

Lemon balm is a powerful antiviral that not only assists our bodies in fighting colds, flus, and cold sore outbreaks but also eases the restlessness that accompanies illness. A tincture, a tea, or a poultice made from fresh or dried leaves provides fast and simple relief for cold sore outbreaks. The first signs of a cold sore might include tingling or swelling at the site before any blistering appears. It is in this critical moment that we begin a medicinal dose of lemon balm: prepare 1 quart of infusion and drink daily. Taken internally it will shorten the life span of the virus and applied externally it will soothe the discomfort of the sore.

HOW IT GROWS

Lemon balm, a member of the mint family, spreads easily and grows abundantly. It loves the sun and under the right conditions can grow up to 3 feet high. I have observed the healthiest, most lemony lemon balm in the sunny summers of the Pacific Northwest. The square stems bear oval, heart-shaped leaves that taper at the end and are bordered with jagged, upward-pointing edges. In late summer, tiny pale yellow, pink, or white flowers appear on the top of the stems in whorls. The leaves are so delightfully lemon scented that merely passing a healthy lemon balm plant will catch your nose. *Melissa* is the Greek word for "bee," so if you hear buzzing and smell something lemony, look down for lemon balm.

TO RECAP

Lemon balm is a popular plant for adults, children, and pollinators. This sour member of the mint family is cooling to hot expressions like cold sores or restless exhaustion. To imagine how something sour could cool you off, think about the popularity of lemonade in the summer months: that "ahhhh" you exhale upon the first sip is the expression of the cooling action of the sour taste.

Cold Sore Ointment

Cold sores are hot, painful, and insecurity inducing. I often get them when I keep putting my needs on the back burner or am too bogged down with responsibility to even remember I have a self. If I catch it too late and the blister grows then I'm really in trouble: uncomfortable and kind of embarrassed. What I need is something to soothe and heal me, physically and emotionally. While it's ideal to have this balm on hand, making it during an outbreak can be a good way to ease back into self-care zone. **Makes two 8-ounce tins.**

SPECIAL EQUIPMENT: JAR OR TINS WITH LIDS

½ cup lemon balm oil

¼ cup licorice oil

¼ cup coconut oil

1 ounce shaved beeswax or beeswax beads

Combine all ingredients in a double boiler over low heat until the beeswax dissolves in the warm oils. Stir to distribute everything evenly. You can pour it all into one large jar or into smaller travel-sized tins. The consistency of this balm is more like an ointment than a traditional lip balm, as the stiffer consistency of a lip balm can tear delicate blisters and irritate sores. Apply with clean hands liberally and often to any outbreaks.

Carmelite Water

Monks and nuns are great resources for medicines that involve alcohol. This recipe is inspired by the water made by Carmelite nuns in the fourteenth century. It's been used as an herbal tonic as well as an eau de toilette back when baths weren't so available or fashionable. If you prefer to avoid alcohol you could prepare this as an infusion and enjoy it over ice cubes on a midsummer's evening. It is gently uplifting and cooling.

Makes 3½ cups.

1 cup fresh lemon balm leaves and tender stems

3 tablespoons dried angelica root

1 tablespoon coriander seed

3 whole cloves

One 4-inch cinnamon stick

6 swipes of nutmeg on a Microplane or fine grater

One 750 ml bottle dry white wine

Combine all the herbs and spices in a glass quart jar. Pour the wine into the jar and stir well (I like to cap it and give it a good shake). I treat mine like a tincture, only I leave it in the refrigerator for 4 to 6 weeks. When you're ready to drink it, strain through a fine-mesh sieve or a few layers of cheesecloth or even a coffee filter. Don't forget to compost the herbs before transferring the infused wine back to the jar. This will keep in the refrigerator for months.

Another option is to make an infused wine with a one-day method. If you start the process in the morning, it can be ready to drink by evening without tasting too much like medicine. You can chill it quickly by wrapping it with a wet towel and putting it in the freezer for 20 minutes before serving. This infused wine should be enjoyed within 3 to 5 days.

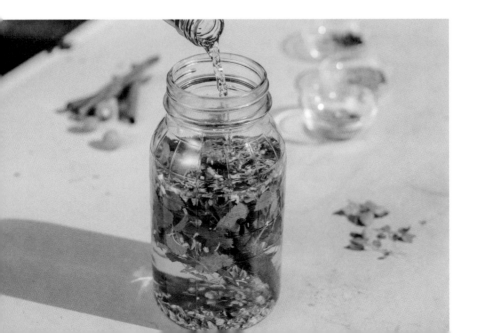

Linden

Tilia spp.

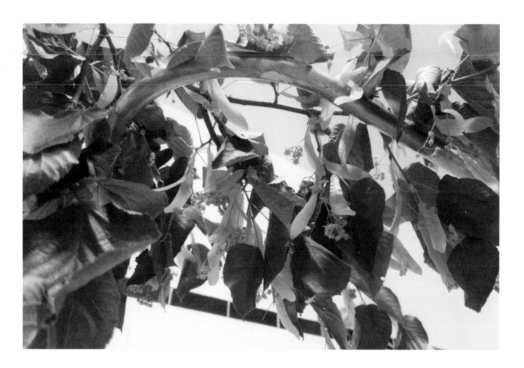

Reach for this when	You need a hug, are feeling anxiety in the form of a racing heart, feel parched and tight, dealing with a virus, feeling restless and anxious
Sensation	Cooling, moist
Flavors	Sweet, mild
Where it lives	A popular street tree abundant in cities and along busy roads
Gather this	Flowers, leaves
Super strengths	Antispasmodic, vasodilator, demulcent, diaphoretic, anti-inflammatory, nervine, cardiotonic

WHY I'M IN LOVE

To behold linden is to swoon. It is, of all these plants, my biggest crush. I could stand for hours under its blooming flowers admiring the bees and enjoying its shade. My teacher Katja Swift calls linden a "hug in a mug." I can't think of a better description of how linden feels in my body or how it feels to stand underneath its elegant limbs and sweet fragrant flowers in June. As someone who tends to run on the dry side, I count on linden to balance the drying effects of plants I rely on daily, like nettle, and those I turn to for special situations, such as hops for when I need extra help going to sleep.

WHAT IT DOES BEST

Linden is a gentle pal. The shade of its limbs adorned with heart-shaped leaves beckons us with the scent of its sweet flowers. That invitation is an offer to uplift and calm. Linden flowers are relaxing to our nervous system: they are particularly helpful when our anxiety manifests in hyperactivity marked by an inability to focus or insomnia. Overtime this kind of anxiety can contribute to tension and tightness in our muscles and cardiovascular system. Linden soothes our tendency to run hot and tight when we're wound up and calms through our circulatory system to relieve tension as it appears as cramps and spasms in our muscles. Linden can help soothe an irritable and wandering mind, gently easing us back into our bodies and our tasks and helping us to unwind so that we may let go of our busy, anxiety-ridden days and experience the restful sleep we need to repair and renew.

When we are feeling blue, linden coaxes us out of certain types of depression. When the thought of someone caring about or for us only aggravates our desire to be left alone, a cup of linden tea can help us find a way toward opening our hearts so that we may let the world in. Even though it hardly ever feels this way when we're deep in it, we are, after all, more likely to feel uplifted in the company of others. But that requires that we get out from under our sheets and out of the house. When we feel like we can't do it alone but can't figure out how to be around other people, linden can wrap us in its embrace and carry us out the door.

If we are sick with a fever and feel hot and thirsty, a warm cup of linden tea can release the frenzied energy of a fever so that our bodies can cool and calm down enough to fight infection. But we don't have to have a fever to benefit from linden's cooling actions. Linden can be like a cool, damp cloth on the back of our necks anytime we feel agitated, especially when our restlessness is fueled by experiences of boredom.

HOW IT GROWS

Linden trees can grow to be 70 feet tall, but I see them in all shapes and sizes. "Lady linden," as I once overhead someone fondly call it, stands confidently in parks and sidewalks, asserting its stately branches and offering the sweet, honeyed perfume scent of its flowers. The heart shape of the leaves can serve as a handy reminder for this plant's affinity for the cardiovascular system. In late spring, the tree develops oblong leaf-like structures called bracts, to which the small yellowish flowers later attach. After the flowers turn to fruit the oblong leaves remain.

TO RECAP

Linden is strong enough to handle the anxiety of being an adult in the world but gentle enough for a child. It soothes and calms feelings of unrest brought on by anxiety, illness, or grief. It is at once calming and moistening, making it appropriate to all situations in which a lot of heat manifests.

Transition Tea

This tea is great for bedtime, when you get off work, or when dealing with loss. Grief can consume us in the wake of loss, at points of transition, or during relocations. It's important to move toward and through these feelings with a lot of support. This tea can help to move the mercurial emotions that show up when we're navigating big life events. **Makes 2 drinks.**

3 cups water

3 teaspoons dried linden flower and leaf

2 teaspoons dried lemon balm

2 teaspoons dried chamomile

Honey

Boil the water, turn off the heat, and let it sit for a couple minutes while you combine the herbs in a teapot. Pour the water over the herbs and let steep for 10 minutes before straining into a mug. Add honey to taste and enjoy warm or over ice.

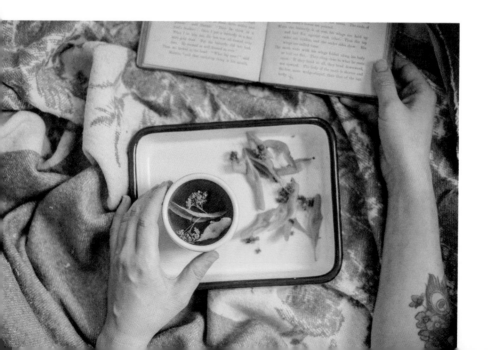

Linden Honey

You can purchase honey made exclusively from linden flowers, but linden also happens to be one of my favorite flowers from which to make a medicinal honey. I like to use both the flower and bract, as it is medicinal. But if you want a stronger-tasting honey, then use only the flowers. Fresh flowers work best for this recipe. **Makes 1½ cups.**

1 cup fresh linden flowers and bracts

1½ cup honey

Fill a glass pint jar with fresh flowers and cover with the honey. Stir to release the air bubbles and make sure the honey coats the plant material. Store in a cool, dark spot for 1 to 4 weeks. Every couple of days or so flip the jar over so the honey and flowers move around. There is no need to strain the honey off the flowers when you're ready to eat some on toast or stir it into a warm drink. Keep the jar in a cool dark place and it will last for a couple of months.

Calming Cubes

These cubes are perfect for a child who's teething or an adult who might be acting like they are. Overtired, restless, and uncomfortable? Take a break with one of these cubes and cool off. If you make these in the morning, which you can do in under 15 minutes, they'll be ready by the time you get home from work or your kid gets home from daycare. **Makes about 25 cubes.**

SPECIAL EQUIPMENT: ICE CUBE TRAYS OR POPSICLE MOLDS AND STICKS

2¾ cups water

⅓ cup Linden Honey (at left, or sugar if you prefer)

2 tablespoons dried chamomile flowers

2 tablespoons dried catnip leaves

2 tablespoons orange blossom water

Boil the water in a small saucepan, turn off the heat, and let it sit for a few seconds. Add the honey, chamomile, and catnip. Cover and steep for 10 minutes. Strain and compost the flowers. Add the orange blossom water to the tea and then fill ice cube trays or popsicle molds leaving a tiny bit of space at the top. If you're making popsicles, place the lid on and insert the sticks. Freeze for at least 8 hours. Run the popsicles under warm water to loosen before taking them out of the mold.

Nettle

Urtica dioica

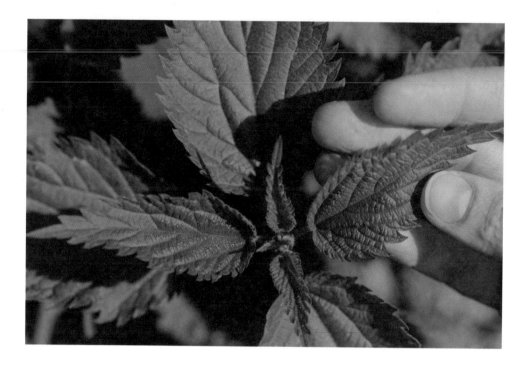

Reach for this when	You're feeling run-down, brain foggy, craving sugar and other processed foods, experiencing seasonal allergies, taking antibiotics, or rebuilding after an illness
Sensation	Cooling, drying
Flavors	Earthy, salty
Where it lives	Wastelands, disturbed earth around barns and near livestock, floodplains, forests edges
Gather this	Leaves, seeds, roots
Super strengths	Nutritive, tonic, tropho-restorative, diuretic, astringent

WHY I'M IN LOVE

I mean really what's not to love? It's one of the first plants that talked to me. No, I am not being hyperbolic—when you spend endless hours with plants outside, in books, and in classrooms you start hearing them. You'll just be minding your own business and all of a sudden you hear "nettle," and you look down, beside you, or up, and there it is, trying to get you to come closer.

Nettle demands that we wake up to our surroundings. It is outfitted with tiny, sharp hairs filled with something like formic acid (the stuff that give ants their sting). When the hairs break and poke into your skin the itchy stuff gets trapped and can stay underneath your skin for days. If you're arthritic, it can bring some relief by ushering blood into the area to move through the stiffness. In the olden days, people used to (and still do) flagellate themselves with the plant for precisely that reason. It's possible to harvest nettle barehanded without getting badly stung, but it requires a lot of awareness and gratitude to interact with a plant in such a way that it can trust you.

WHAT IT DOES BEST

Since it's kind of the elephant in the room I'll just say it: our modern industrialized diet sucks. It's not totally our fault, but we can take the direction of our health into our own hands. Nettle is the go-to plant among herbalists. Everyone can benefit from it, because we all live in a modern world where we are surrounded by environmental pollution, allergens, toxicity, and systemic oppression. As a densely nutritious diuretic, nettle ramps up your health by sweeping out waste and ushering in vitamins and minerals that help your body replenish and recover from the demands of modern life. It is high in chlorophyll, protein, vitamins A, K, and lots of the Bs, iron, calcium, and trace minerals like selenium and zinc. Because all parts of nettle are so chock-full of good-for-us stuff it can quickly overhaul your health in a serious way.

HOW IT GROWS

Nettle spreads similarly to mint, grows in every state except Arkansas (according to the USDA), and appears in early spring. From its squarish, hairy stem, simple, usually opposite leaves, grow. The leaves are toothed with stinging hairs on the underside. The older plants can grow to 5 feet and produce strong fibers from which bed linens and clothes are made. For this reason the younger leaves toward the top of the plant are better suited to eating.

TO RECAP

A favorite plant of many herbalists, nettle is appropriate under most circumstances and constitutions. For constitutions that are already hot and dry, nettle's drying tendency can be easily offset by the addition of linden leaf and flower, violet leaf, or marshmallow root.

The more nourished we are, the better our whole body functions and the more capable we are in handling stressful conditions. That's where nettle comes in. Nettle is an excellent source of trace minerals. "Trace" refers to tiny amounts of minerals we need that are stored in our body. They include things like iron, zinc, fluoride, iodine, copper, selenium, and manganese. Trace minerals are essential minerals that help the body perform vital functions. For example, we need them to rebalance a stressed-out body and mind. The perfect storm of stress in modern life can have us running on reserves, which is definitely not sustainable. One way we experience stress is through what's called perceived stress, not because it may or may not exist, but because it changes from person to person. Some examples include allergies to pollen or pets, working too much, and being targeted by oppression. Over time chronic stress can show up as eczema outbreaks, brain fog, and feeling burnt out. The seed of nettle in particular can improve our energy level and promote clarity so that we can move through the brain fog to help us make better choices in supporting good health.

Nourishing Infusion

Once the first signs of spring start to sprout I go hard on the nettle infusion. A quart of nettle infusion per day—yes, every day—means a lot of support for our endocrine system, which includes our adrenal glands. As we move into a season that requires more energy output—we move more, start to eat raw foods again, and many of our bodies battle allergies—nettles can help support our stamina and energy levels. Nettles can be drying so I like to combine them with some moistening plants and others that are appropriate for the transition into spring. **Makes 4 cups.**

½ cup nettle leaves

¼ cup red clover flowers

¼ cup calendula flowers

1 tablespoon marshmallow root

2 tablespoons peppermint leaves

Combine all herbs in a bowl and divide evenly between 2 quart-sized jars, fill with just boiled water, cap lightly (I just use the round disk insert that comes as part of Ball jar lids), and let it infuse on the counter for 30 minutes before refrigerating for 8 hours. I like to prepare my infusion at night, so that I wake up to an inky green, life-affirming drink! The moistening action of marshmallow root activates in cold water but if you prefer to drink room temp or warm beverages adding warm water won't mess up the demulcent effects of the infusion.

If you intend to eat or make tea from nettle leaves, do so before the plant flowers. While you can safely harvest and consume the seed in the late summer and early fall, the cystoliths that develop in mature plants may potentially contribute to kidney and liver damage. Play it safe and stick to eating young growth in the spring and early summer before the plant flowers.

Nutrient Dust

Nutrient dust is a vitamin-packed condiment that I keep within arm's reach of my stove. Add this savory salt to cooked rice, sautéed vegetables, or popcorn. Throw a handful in the soup you're making or mix it into a salad dressing. You can eat it on anything and every part of your body will thank you for it.

Besides nettle, nutrient dust contains sea vegetables (kelp and dulse). Brown and green seaweeds are essential to our daily intake of iodine and to carrying out toxins that accumulate in our bodies. I like to buy seaweed from Maine Seaweed, LLC. It is important to buy from people who harvest from clean waters and who harvest sustainably as stewards, not just resource-suckers. **Makes about 1 cup.**

3 large kelp strips
½ cup dried nettle parts
¼ cup dulse flakes

I like to toast the kelp for this recipe. Preheat the oven to 375°F, distribute the kelp strips on a baking sheet in a single layer, and toast for around 10 minutes, until the kelp goes from green to toasty brown. Let the seaweed cool to room temperature. Combine the kelp, nettle, and dulse flakes in a food processor or blender and pulse until everything is the size of flaky salt (or use a mortar and pestle). Store at room temperature out of direct sunlight.

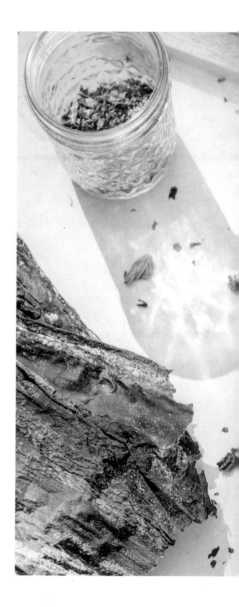

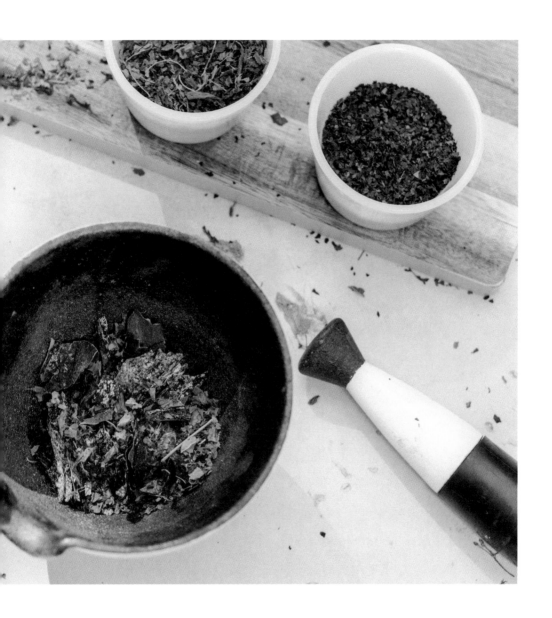

Peppermint

Mentha × piperita

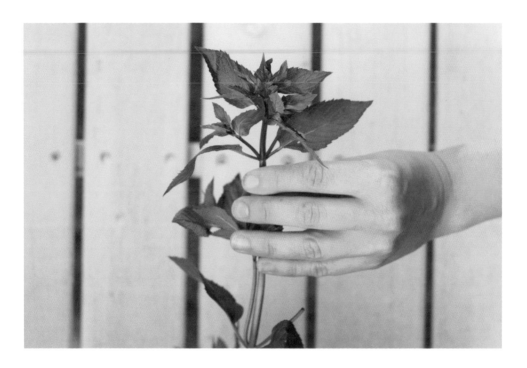

Reach for this when	You seek invigorating refreshment, you've got a stomach situation that needs soothing, you've got to do some cleaning
Sensation	Cooling, drying, refreshing, invigorating, comforting
Flavors	Sweet, aromatic, pungent
Where it lives	Cool, damp places, bits of sun
Gather this	Leaves, flowers
Super strengths	Antispasmodic, carminative, antimicrobial, antifungal, stimulant, relaxant, analgesic

WHY I'M IN LOVE

Collectively, we love the taste of peppermint. It's in our chocolates, ice cream, gum, and toothpaste. More than the taste though, is the feeling of peppermint: the cool refreshment that at once invigorates and calms. I can't help but think of the Ice Breakers gum commercials featuring a white unicorn bounding through imagined winter, blasting through walls of ice. The sensation of peppermint breaks through to release whatever is in the way. Peppermint bestows new strength with which to move through moments of tension.

WHAT IT DOES BEST

If you're in your midthirties, and for example, made the mistake of overindulging (say a cocktail, a beer, a glass of wine, or a generous serving of dessert all in the name of fun), and find yourself pulling the covers over your eyes to mollify the demands of the early Saturday morning sunlight, peppermint can be just the ticket to emerge from the darkness. The aroma of a simple infusion of peppermint leaves or a few drops of peppermint essential oil diluted in a carrier oil like jojoba, almond, or sesame and applied to the temples relieves tension headaches caused by things like too much sugar.

Peppermint is especially skilled at keeping potentially embarrassing inconveniences at bay. It makes a superb digestive aid when sipped after a meal, because it relieves gas and bloating. While peppermint is commonly regarded as relaxing, this action points to its stimulating effects in the body: it calms by moving. Its stimulating effects can also be useful when fighting illness, as part of peppermint's work is to speed things along. Even though the menthol in peppermint tricks the receptors on our tongue and skin into thinking we're cold, internally it lights a bit of a fire under the processes in our bodies that can get periodically or chronically sluggish, tired, and tight. This is the action of refreshment: assisting our bodies in the demands to constantly restrengthen, reinvigorate, and renew.

HOW IT GROWS

Once peppermint starts growing, it is unlikely to stop. As a mint it sprawls, so it's a great plant for containers like window boxes and small indoor pots. It grows happily and bushily in small spaces. Its purplish square stems bear opposite leaves. The deep green leaves get darker through the summer, bordering on purple toward the fall when light purple flowers appear in whorls at the tip of the stem. It can get quite high in the dog days of summer, reaching up to 1½ feet tall. The more you pick it, the more it will grow, showcasing its own resiliency and generosity with each pluck.

TO RECAP

Peppermint is a refreshing, renewing, rejuvenating blast to our system. It can help us feel energized without demanding that we overexert ourselves. It is my favorite plant for headache relief, especially one related to too much junk food or alcohol.

Four Thieves All-Purpose Cleaner

Legend has it this aromatic vinegar kept four French thieves free of the bubonic plague while they robbed the bodies of the dead. There are many recipes and lots of speculation as to how, why, and if it actually worked. I do know it makes an effective all-purpose cleaner that doesn't hurt the environment when it goes down the drain. Traditionally garlic is included in the preparation that's meant to be ingested, but I leave it out when I'm making a batch for cleaning. **Makes about 4 cups.**

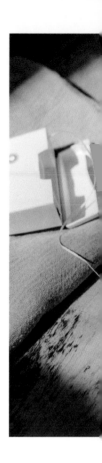

2 tablespoons fresh mint leaves, chopped

2 tablespoons fresh rosemary leaves and soft stems, chopped

2 tablespoons fresh sage leaves, chopped

2 tablespoons fresh oregano leaves, chopped

2 tablespoons fresh lavender flowers, chopped

Peel of 2 lemons

2 tablespoons dried clove, roughly chopped

3 cinnamon sticks, broken into smaller pieces

4 cups white distilled vinegar

Combine everything in a 2-quart jar, cap with a plastic lid or a metal lid lined with plastic wrap. Shake thoroughly and store in a cool place out of direct sunlight. Remember to shake every few days for the next 6 weeks and up to 3 months. Strain and compost the solids, then pour the infused vinegar into a spray bottle. It's great on windows and glass, cuts grease, and cleans bathrooms!

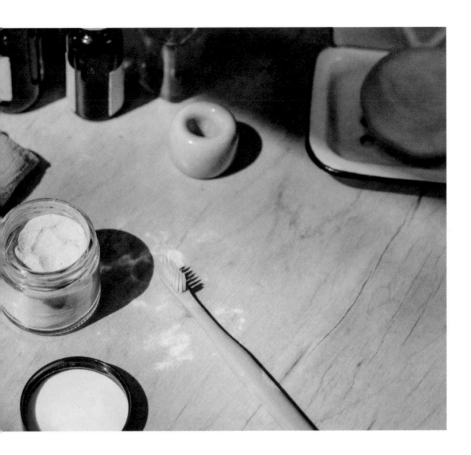

Peppermint-Fresh Toothpowder

Peppermint is listed as the active ingredient in most toothpastes and is advertised as doing the work of cleaning our teeth, but in reality, it just produces an exciting feeling in our mouths and on our tongues. Peppermint flavor itself doesn't actually clean our mouths, but it makes it *feel* like it does. I like to make a little powder for traveling as it is easy to use, does the trick, isn't a big deal if I swallow some of it, doesn't require a lot of water, and leaves my mouth feeling refreshed. **Makes about ½ cup.**

1 tablespoon baking soda

¼ cup powdered bentonite clay

2 tablespoons dried ground peppermint

½ teaspoon dried ground clove

1 teaspoon fine sea salt

Combine all ingredients in a small bowl and stir. I like to store my toothpowder in a shallow airtight tub and use my fingers to sprinkle it on my toothbrush. Brush away.

Red Clover

Trifolium pratense

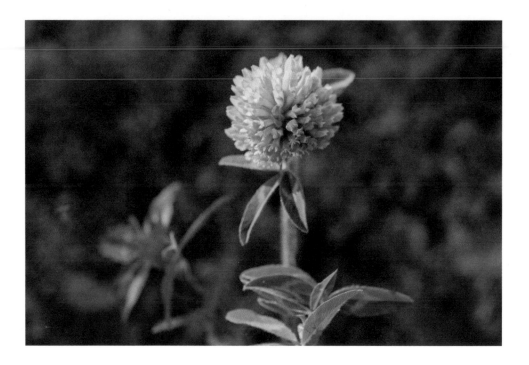

Reach for this when	Your skin or eyes feel dry and irritated, you've undergone a course of antibiotics, you have dry, swollen glands
Sensation	Cool, moist
Flavors	Sweet
Where it lives	Pastures, orchards, highway medians
Gather this	Flowers
Super strengths	Alterative, antispasmodic, nutritive, tonic, expectorant, lymphagogue

WHY I'M IN LOVE

Dense blankets of red clover's bright pink flower heads dance over fields of green bordering two lane highways in the towns I frequent in upstate New York. Their fuzzy heads, which resemble fireworks, bob in the wind and stretch in the heat of the late summer sun. I also see them popping up in apple orchards or in sunny, forgotten patches of suburban or country yards. You don't need more than a few flower heads to make a quick cooling drink to sip in the afternoon sun. It's nutritive and soothing and it goes great with wandering around barefoot while you wait for the sun to set.

WHAT IT DOES BEST

If I'm looking to get a little bit more out of red clover, then I'll let the flowers work their magic in water overnight. As I rest, water-soluble vitamins and minerals like vitamins A, C, E, and K, calcium, magnesium, and potassium, plus protein infuse the water and in the morning I have a super drink! I like to drink red clover infused with other helpful plants at least once a week, or more if I'm experiencing dryness in or on my body.

Red clover is also wonderfully moistening and is an excellent remedy for dry, unproductive coughs. Its antispasmodic action cools and relaxes airways and lungs, soothing irritation in your respiratory system.

Another telltale sign that I need red clover is when dry patches develop on my face or the corners of my eyes feel parched. Anytime our skin suffers, something is most likely happening a bit below the surface. Many skin conditions can be traced back to a sluggish lymphatic system. Red clover helps remove congestion in the lymphatic system after wastes accumulate in the wake of an illness, especially after a course of antibiotics or when we've been riding the sugar, alcohol, or caffeine train kind of hard. This, in turn, improves the quality of our blood, clearing away eczema and other skin irritations characterized by dryness or cracking. Taken internally as a nourishing infusion or applied externally as a poultice, red clover is soothing to dry, irritated skin.

HOW IT GROWS

Red clover is a perennial that prefers fields and meadows. The characteristic purple-pink flower blooms on a separate stalk from the root. The stalks are hairy and bear slightly obovate, trifoliate leaves, most of which are marked with a white or light green chevron in the upper middle third of the leaf.

TO RECAP

Red clover is both soothing and mildly activating to sluggishness in our bodies. It gently relaxes as it provides us with vitamins and minerals.

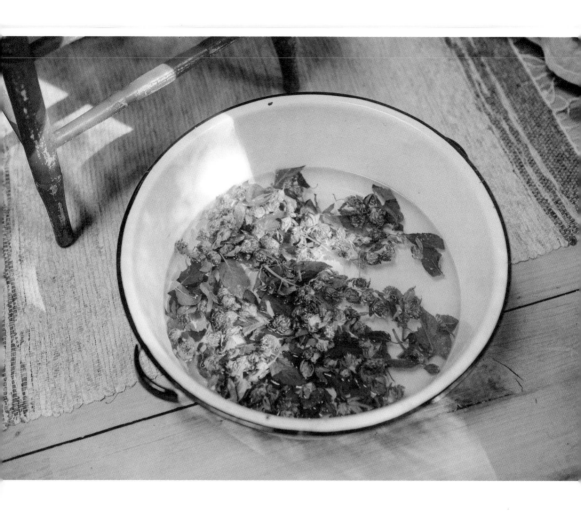

Foot Bath

I am on my feet 8 hours a day for most of the week. This simple foot soak not only alleviates the heavy, leaden feeling in my legs, but relaxes me with its aromas of thyme and mint. **Makes enough for 1 bath.**

2 cups fresh red clover blossoms

1 cup chopped fresh peppermint leaves and flowers

Handful chopped fresh thyme leaves and flowers

8 cups water

Fill a basin with the herbs and boil the water. Pour the water over the herbs and allow the water to infuse while you wait for it to be a suitable temperature. Grab a book or queue up a podcast and take a load off.

Iced Tea

When my friend Cyd picks me up at the train station upstate she reports on the healthfulness of her red clover population. She has a beautifully kept garden and an equally pleasing wildness to her yard. I like to wander around her property barefoot and pop the blossoms off red clover plants to make us a simple infusion to enjoy with a sprig of peppermint and a squeeze of lemon over ice. **Makes 3½ cups.**

2 dozen fresh red clover blossoms

4 cups hot water

Boil the water, turn off the heat, and let it cool for a few minutes. Put the blossoms in a glass quart jar or teapot and pour over the water. Let it infuse for at least 20 minutes and up to 12 hours before straining. I like to do this either early in the morning or in the evening while the sun sets. This way I am guaranteed tea in time for a post-lunch lounge on Cyd's dock.

Rose

Rosa spp.

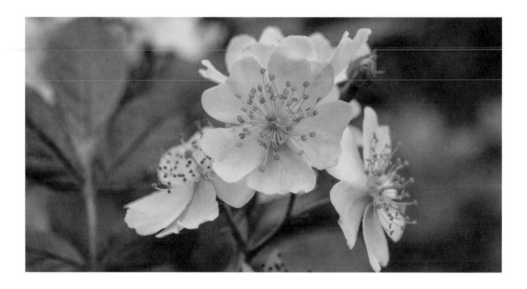

Reach for this when	Hips: you're in the mood for some vitamin C, preparing red meat, in need of a mild laxative
	Petals: you need to cool off in a big way, are having a hard time recalling the sweet parts of life, burned yourself, working on vulnerability
Sensation	Hips: neutral (not as cooling as petals, but still on the cool side), drying
	Petals: cooling, drying
Flavors	Hips: sweet, sour
	Petals: sweet, mildly bitter
Where it lives	Cultivated gardens, bordering sunny paths on the edge of woods and fields, prefers some shade and some sun
Gather this	Petals, leaves, hips, stems, and even the "thorns" (actually prickles)
Super strengths	Antispasmodic, anti-inflammatory, nervine, astringent, nutritive, antioxidant, carminative, cardiotonic, laxative (rose hips)

WHY I'M IN LOVE

All parts of rose are wound healing: from external wounds to internal wounds to emotional wounds. I rely on rose to cool sunburns, relieve a burned tongue when I bite into a pizza that hasn't cooled yet, or when I can feel frustration welling up inside me like a fire, building and desperately searching for ways to release. Rose has a habit of calming and cooling me down, especially when those feelings of burning are paired with vulnerability.

WHAT IT DOES BEST

Rose petals are maybe most commonly known as an aphrodisiac. Lead your lover to bed with petals, scatter them in a sexy bath, feed them to the linen swans on your honeymoon bed. It's an aphrodisiac because it's an excellent blood mover: it gets things going and opens the heart up. This is not to be confused with heating things up; that's what ginger does. Rose is a mover because it is calming and imparts feelings of safety and protection. Consider a small animal, perhaps a rabbit, who finds shelter and protection in the cool shade of a rose bush. Fleeing a predator, she scurries beneath the prickled, rambling branches where it's cool, sweet-scented, and quiet. This is the gift of rose: an aromatic, cool, shaded moment of rest. A place to breathe, to collect oneself, and plan what's next. The physical and emotional come together and enable us to be vulnerable enough to love, have sex without so much anxiety, or just be in the company of others with more ease. Turn to rose petals to help you open your heart and let someone or something in.

Rose hips are harvested in autumn: they are high in vitamin C and pectin, so they make excellent jams or savory tapenades for fall and winter roasts of meat. Like the petals, hips are also high in bioflavonoids—one of the things that give plants their color and antioxidant properties.

HOW IT GROWS

Multiflora rose self-seeds and spreads easily. When the U.S. Soil Conservation Service encouraged its use as an effective control for erosion during the 1930s, they had no idea it would be so invasive. Like other members of the rose family, its petals grow in clusters of five. The petals are white and grow wider the further they are from the stamen. Rose plants grow bushy and hedge-like, bumping up against fences with branches that reach and curl to form dense thickets. I've seen bushes bordering highways in upstate New York that push 15 feet. The branches and stems are covered in prickles, which, like thorns, are a leaf adaptation.

TO RECAP

Because rose medicine is generally needed immediately—to soothe a temper, comfort someone in the wake of some kind of trauma, or ease a broken heart—it's nice to have dried rose petals on hand. A situation that begs for a cup of rose tea could come out of nowhere and you'll be happy you were prepared.

Rose Petal Toast

Rose is welcome any time of day in my house. But petals on bread is particularly delicious as a pre-breakfast or late afternoon snack with iced tea in the summer. Planning a day hike? Take along everything but the roses and hope that you find some bordering your walking path. Be sure to choose a piece of nice bread. I like something kind of dense but sweet, like a bread with oatmeal. If it's fresh I don't bother toasting it because I like the crunchy crust and the soft interior. **Serves 1.**

1 tablespoon (or more! Personally I like the kind of butter spread that leaves toothmarks after a bite) delicious cultured butter, the yellower the better

1 thick slice of fresh baked bread

1 tablespoon honey

Fresh edible rose petals (from about 4 wild roses that have not been chemically treated or sprayed with pesticides)

Generous pinch of flaky salt

Slather a thick layer of butter on the bread, drizzle with a bit of honey, sprinkle the petals on top, and finish with flaky salt.

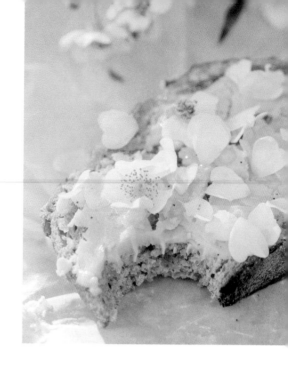

Burn Spray

This cheery, cooling little bottle of pink magic never leaves my side when the sun is high and hot in the sky. **Makes about 1 cup.**

1 cup edible rose petals

1 cup apple cider vinegar

Follow the directions for making an Herbal Vinegar Hair Rinse (page 169) using rose petals. After straining off the rose petals, fill a 2-ounce spray bottle a third of the way up with the rose vinegar and fill the rest with distilled water (In a pinch I just let some tap water sit out overnight so the chlorine evaporates). Bring your bottle to the beach to refresh your skin after an afternoon in the salt and sun. Do not spray this on a red, blistered burn—it will feel terrible.

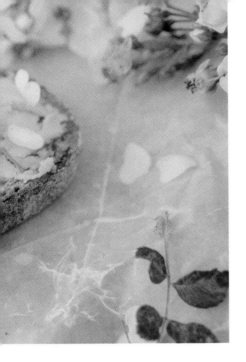

Face Mask

The easiest way to incorporate more healthy habits into our lives is by sneaking them in during routines we've already established. Most of us have a bedtime routine that helps us wind down and shift into snooze-gear. Occasionally it's nice to prolong this small window of self-love by applying a face mask. I love this mask for its cleansing and moisturizing properties, but what I find most exciting is the magical transformation that happens when I hydrate it with rose water before slathering it on: it turns instantly from gray to pink! **Makes about 15 face masks.**

2 tablespoons rolled oats
⅓ cup dried rose petals
2 tablespoons bentonite clay
Rose water

Grind the oats and rose petals in a spice grinder until they form a fine powder. Combine them with the bentonite clay in a bowl. Store the dry face mask in an airtight container. When you're ready for some pampering, put a heaping teaspoon of the powder mix in a bowl and add enough rose water to form a thick-but-wet paste. Apply the mask to your face and sit back for 15 to 20 minutes while it dries. Rinse and follow with an application of your Cooling Eye Balm (page 113).

The rose family is vast with thousands of varieties, which can be pretty over-whelming at first glance. Depending on where you are in the world, country, or state, you might hear different names for the same rose or the same name for different roses. These names can shift across geographic lines, among different ethnic groups, and even over time. The wild rose or "species rose" is a true wildflower with no help from humans. The photographs illustrate the multiflora rose, a white variety origi-nally from Japan that was planted as a living fence by upstate New Yorkers in the early twentieth century. It is now *everywhere*. It is considered a noxious weed in some states, threatening native populations because of its prolific seed production as well as harboring rose rosette virus, which is bad news for cultivated roses.

Rosemary

Rosmarinus officinalis

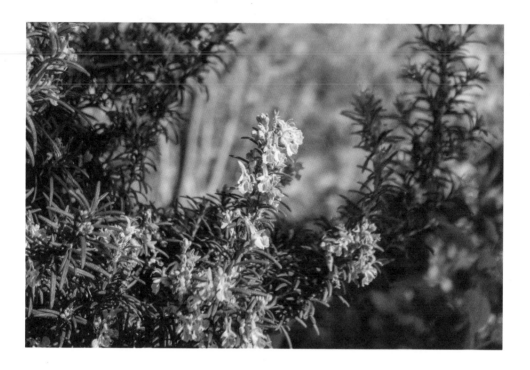

Reach for this when	You need a gently stimulating pick-me-up, are cooking meat (especially red meat), are experiencing trouble focusing
Sensation	Warming, drying, sticky
Flavors	Pungent, spicy
Where it lives	Native to the Mediterranean, it loves sun and abhors soggy soil; it prefers rocky, even "bad," soil and can stand up to pretty harsh conditions
Gather this	Leaves, twigs, flowers
Super strengths	Antioxidant, aromatic, carminative, circulatory stimulant, antimicrobial, nervine, hepatic, relaxant, cardiotonic

WHY I'M IN LOVE

I keep a small potted rosemary plant near my desk. When I'm sitting down to do something that gives me anxiety and having trouble concentrating I clip a sprig, rub it between my hands, and breathe. Rosemary's scent brings me a calming clarity, similar to how I feel after dunking in the Atlantic. But since I live in the middle of Brooklyn the quickest way to the sea is through rosemary. If you happen to adore the ocean like me, then the translation of rosemary's Latin name—"dew of the sea"—might resonate with you. To swim and splash in the sea feels restorative. Like the ocean, rosemary quiets the spots that are humming too loudly or too often and invigorates those that have grown dull.

WHAT IT DOES BEST

Any place in our body or our lives that has slowed down, stopped, or clenched is a good spot for rosemary. Its warming actions are stimulating to our scalp, heart, digestive system, muscles, and minds. Every once in a while, I replace store-bought conditioners with a simple infusion of rosemary in apple cider vinegar (see page 169) and now my hair grows longer and my scalp is less dry and itchy. The volatile oils stimulate hair growth and reduce dandruff. Rosemary moves blood throughout our body to reach places that could benefit from movement and a sense of opening. It acts as a crucial tonic for the heart by gently increasing circulation and decreasing inflammation. These actions extend to other muscles in our bodies. Say,

for example, you were up late watching old Richard Simmons clips and then decide to join that outdoor boot camp you always see on Saturday mornings when you're going to the bagel shop to nurse your hangover. So anyway, after weeks or months of doing minimal activity, in one morning you do a million squats and bench press your trainer, because you were so jazzed. The next day your body will be calling out for a rosemary-infused oil to relax and soothe sore muscles that have seized and stiffened from too much too soon. Arthritic or wounded parts of our bodies where we experience pain with inflammation can also be eased with rosemary.

I can't think of rosemary without wanting prime rib; it's a classic pairing for good reason. Rosemary appears alongside so many meat dishes because it supports the liver and assists in digestion of the fats, easing digestive complaints like gas and heaviness that accompany rich meals.

HOW IT GROWS

Rosemary is an evergreen in the mint family so under the right conditions it can really flourish. In parts of the Pacific Northwest, I've seen 6-foot-high towering shrubs teeming with bees and delivering a jolt of energy as you walk by. Lower parts of rosemary are woody, higher up are more flexible, green stems that support fresh growth. The tops of the plant are adorned with purple flowers in spring and summer.

Many people are fond of hanging eucalyptus branches in their bathrooms. I prefer rosemary because it's less expensive and more invigorating. In my tendency to get distracted and then feel guilty, rosemary keeps me from descending into a blame spiral that can end in zero concentration, or worse, bouts of depression. It helps me feel calm and reminds me to keep moving so I don't get stuck in places that hold me back or bring me down. This can be particularly helpful in the morning, awakening and brightening my day before I have a chance to bog myself down with negativity or self-doubt.

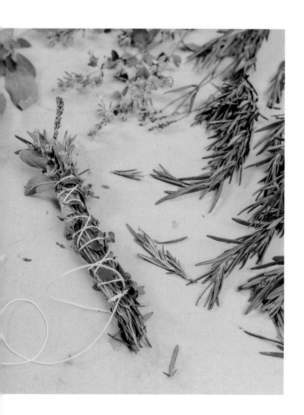

Incense

Lots of us are burning things we really shouldn't: many popular smudges are made from sacred, at-risk plants like white sage and palo santo. If you aren't a member of the communities who have special relationships with these plants, it might be time to stop burning them. The good news is that plants come from all over the world just like people, so you too probably have a more appropriate plant somewhere in your ancestry! Mine happens to be rosemary. I make incense bundles from rosemary and other popular garden or farm plants like lavender and garden sage. A simple aromatic incense can help clear the air and free our minds so we can focus on taking care of ourselves and each other. **Makes 3 bundles.**

1 bunch fresh rosemary
1 bunch fresh lavender
1 bunch fresh garden sage

I like to start with a few good sturdy stalks of rosemary and then add one or two of the other plants, wrapping them around to make a loose herb wand. Then, wrap kitchen twine a few times around the base, leaving a little tail that you'll use later to tie off the twine. Continue to wrap as you move up the bundle and then back down to make a crisscross pattern with the twine, tying off at the base and snipping the twine. Repeat with the remaining herbs to make additional bundles. Hang the bundles upside down to dry in an airy place out of direct sunlight. They should be ready in about 2 weeks, depending on the humidity.

Focus Tea

This tea is a perfect companion for studying or reading especially on a cloudy day or when you need just a little bit of a kick in the evening but definitely don't want caffeine.
Makes 3 cups.

¼ cup roughly chopped fresh rosemary leaves and twigs

½ orange, sliced ¼-inch thick

½ Meyer lemon, sliced ¼-inch thick

3 cups hot water

Honey

Combine the rosemary, orange, and lemon in a teapot and cover with the water. Let steep for 7 to 10 minutes before straining. Pour into a mug and stir in honey to taste and enjoy.

Weekend Bath Salts

After a long week, do yourself a favor by taking a hot bath with Epsom salts and invigorating herbs: it relaxes the body, gets blood moving through the legs, and calms the mind after hectic weekdays. **Makes about 8 cups.**

Peels of 3 lemons

5 cups Epsom salts

2 cups dried rosemary leaves

¼ cup whole cloves

First, dry your lemon peel. Use a peeler to make wide strips of lemon peel and then slice them crosswise into ¼-inch-thick strips. Spread them in a single layer on a piece of parchment paper or plate and let them dry for about 3 days. Once dry you can continue with assembling the rest of the bath salts.

Put the dried peels, salt, rosemary, and cloves in a big bowl and stir together, then transfer to two wide-mouthed quart jars or other appropriately sized vessels. When you're ready to take a bath, fill a muslin bag with 1 cup of the salt blend and sling it over the faucet so the water runs over and through the salt and herbs on its way into the tub. Tap water transformed into spa water before your eyes!

Herbal Vinegar Hair Rinse

Makes about 2 cups.

½ cup fresh rosemary leaves

¼ cup dried calendula flowers

¼ cup dried lavender flowers

2 cups apple cider vinegar

Combine the herbs and flowers in a pint jar and cover with the apple cider vinegar. Cap with a plastic lid or a metal lid lined with plastic wrap. Place in a cool, dark place for 2 to 4 weeks, then strain and compost the plant solids.

To use, apply two tablespoons of the vinegar to damp hair, massage it into the scalp, and then rinse thoroughly. If your scalp is so dry that it is raw or cracked in places, do not apply vinegar. Your rinse will last about a year stored in a cool, dark place.

Staghorn Sumac

Rhus typhina

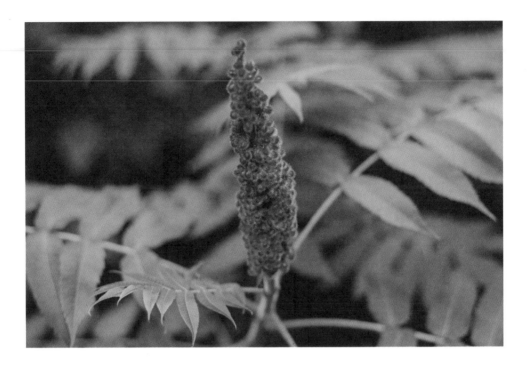

Reach for this when	You can't stop sweating, you have diarrhea, you're in the first few days of your menstrual cycle, or in the middle or wake of a stressful event or time of your life
Sensation	Cooling, drying
Flavors	Sour
Where it lives	Bordering highways, meadows on the edge of forests, backyards from Mexico to Canada
Gather this	Bark, fruit/berries
Super strengths	Carminative, hepatic, astringent, diuretic, antiseptic, antimicrobial, antioxidant, antifungal, anti-inflammatory, tonic, relaxant, nutritive

WHY I'M IN LOVE

When I was little we would drive from New Jersey to Florida to visit my grandparents. As we drove deeper and deeper into the South I loved rolling down my window to let in the damp, hot air. Reaching over highway walls and sprawling behind chain link fences were these beautiful, bushy trees with fuzzy branches and burgundy horns poking through the feathery leaves. If I had paid an ounce more attention to my natural world where I lived, I would have noticed the unmistakable staghorn of the sumac tree almost everywhere. It's helpful that my memories place one of my favorite trees in an environment to which it offers the perfect relief: the thick heavy southern heat. Sumac is abundant and scrappy, showing up almost everywhere and anywhere to help us keep cool and dry.

WHAT IT DOES BEST

Sumac is one of the best plants to allay overheating and profuse sweating, plus it's full of antioxidants. At a certain point, sweat, or any fluid loss for that matter, can feel like uncomfortable oozing: it seems to come from everywhere and is difficult to stop. We can lose water in lots of ways: sweating, peeing often, or from diarrhea. Sumac is especially helpful in situations where fear or nervousness is driving these responses. Sumac gently cleanses and tones so that we can hang on to liquids that we need and stop excessive leaking, so to speak. In the process it provides vitamin C so that our bodies can repair or make new connective tissue,

like our skin and blood vessels. Sumac's high antioxidant presence protects cells from free radicals.

Not only a summer medicine, sumac works wonders in the winter as well. Drippy head colds characterized by wet sneezes, wet lungs, and postnasal drip are no match for sumac. While the deeper airways are generally ideal locations to host a virus, sumac helps to literally dry up our naturally hospitable environment to viruses. If you have the type of cold that sends you into a coughing fit the moment you rest your head, sumac might be an appropriate remedy.

HOW IT GROWS

Sumac is a sight to behold year round. The tree bears tender, toothed, green leaves in spring. Early summer spawns white flowers that are popular with bees. Toward the end of June the unmistakable burgundy horns begin to grow: green at first with flecks of pink that deepen as the summer goes on until they turn deep burgundy in early summer and are ready for harvesting. It is best to harvest the berries before they dry if you don't want to deal with worms. They can be stripped from the cone, washed and dried, or tinctured fresh to enjoy throughout the year. In winter, sumac's skeletal limbs support the fuzzy horns of berries known as sumac bobs; the dried fruit is a reliable food source for wild turkeys and other birds through the long winter. While sumac is technically a shrub, I have seen some trees that tower over 20 feet high. It can tolerate harsh soil conditions and the intensity of locations such as highways so we often see it there because it also effectively controls erosion. It is prolific in North America, with native and non-native species growing in the deserts of Mexico, all of the United States, and in every province in Canada.

TO RECAP

Sumac can help us deal with some of the consequences of high-anxiety modern life. Coupled with stress fighters like tulsi and calming plants like chamomile or lemon balm, it can help to ease our system back into a state of relaxation and repair. Its astringent qualities tone the muscles and soft tissues in our bodies that experience inflammation in the wake of a stressful event. It is the perfect beverage to sip in the heat of late August. Making tea gives us a moment to pause and relax with an ice cold beverage in the breeze, if we're lucky enough to find any.

Sumac Coolie

This is my favorite deep-summer drink for after exercising, at the beach, and during picnics. You can sweeten it with honey, sugar, or nothing at all. When I don't want to add any sweetener I'll include some cinnamon chips to give it a little sweet kick. **Makes 8 cups.**

Berries from 3 sumac bobs (fresh or dried)
½ cup hibiscus flowers
¼ cup rose petals
2 tablespoons cinnamon chips (optional)
Honey or sugar (optional)

Add the sumac berries, hibiscus, rose, and cinnamon chips, if desired, to a 2-quart jar and fill halfway with just boiled water. Steep for 15 minutes, then add your sweetener to taste, if desired, as it will incorporate better while the infusion is still warm. Fill the jar with ice cubes. As the liquid cools the ice melts and makes the perfect tea for drinking even colder over ice. It's even delicious with a little vodka or tequila.

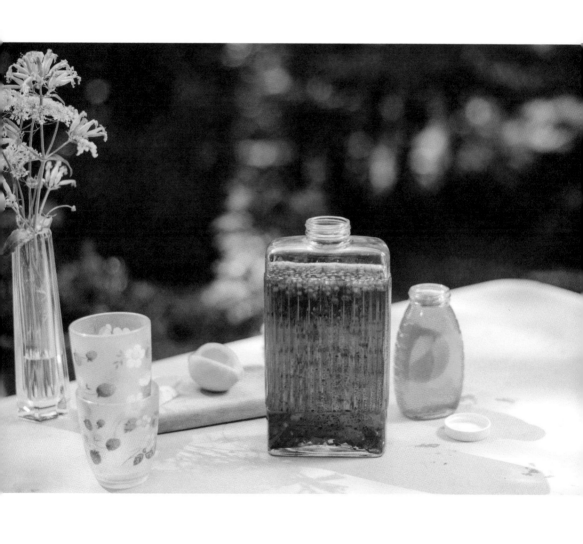

Sumac Spice

To make sumac spice, harvest fresh sumac bobs early in the season as soon as the berries reach full burgundy. The earlier you get to them, the less likely you'll be fighting with worms and molds. It's not as easy as going to the store, but the fruits of your labor will be tasty, rewarding, and long-lasting. **Yield varies on harvest.**

SPECIAL EQUIPMENT: DEHYDRATOR

Fresh sumac bobs

Rinse the bobs and then dry them in a dehydrator at 125°F for 10 hours or in an oven on low for 2 to 5 hours. When dry, strip the berries into a blender, buzz until everything is a mess, and push everything through a fine-mesh sieve to separate the spice from the seeds. Discard the seeds. Stored out of direct light and heat, sumac spice will keep for at least 1 year.

Za'atar

Years ago my friends brought back za'atar from Palestine: it was the most vibrant green and smelled richly of the aromatic spices that give it its characteristic taste. Sumac is a key ingredient in this popular Middle Eastern spice blend. Try sprinkling it on yogurt, grilled vegetables, toasted pita or sourdough, eggs, or avocados. It also makes a tasty spice rub for meats. **Makes about ½ cup.**

2 tablespoons Sumac Spice (at left)
2 tablespoons dried oregano leaf
2 tablespoons dried thyme leaf
2 tablespoons toasted sesame seeds
2 teaspoons kosher salt

Combine the sumac spice, oregano, and thyme in a mortar and pestle and apply gentle but steady pressure to mix and meld the flavors of the plants together. Transfer to an airtight container and mix in the sesame seeds and salt. Store with your herbs and spices, discard after a year.

Staghorn sumac is in the same botanical family as poison sumac but the two are not related. Poison sumac is more closely related to poison ivy and oaks than to other sumacs. Poison sumac is distinguishable from other sumacs by its leaflets, which are not saw-toothed or fuzzy, but long, ovate, and smooth. Where staghorn sumac's red berries grow upward in a cone shape, the white berries of poison sumac hang from the branches, more like grapes than a horn. Without leaves or berries you can identify poison sumac by its red stems. It also grows in wetlands, and by wetlands I mean it grows in so much water that other trees around it are likely dead from the excess. While it is not wise to walk out your front door and go grazing on anything that resembles viable food, it is also unwise to live in fear of all plants just because they have a similar name. Plants *are* distinguishable from one another, we have entire fields of study based on this truth, and it is your responsibility to learn how to identify plants with 100 percent certainty.

Thyme

Thymus vulgaris

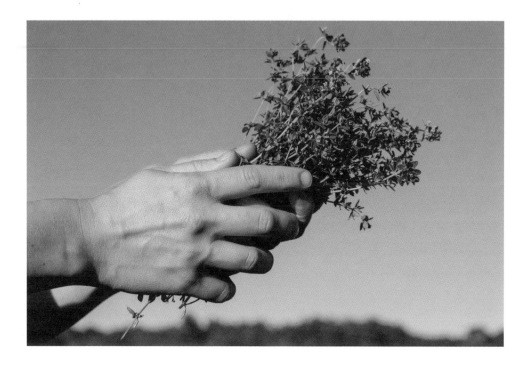

Reach for this when	You have a wet cough, a sore throat, you're getting ready to eat, you need to deeply calm yourself
Sensation	Dry, hot
Flavors	Pungent, spicy
Where it lives	Mostly in cultivated gardens, in dry, sandy soil
Gather this	Leaves and flowers
Super strengths	Diaphoretic, stimulating relaxant, antimicrobial, nervine, expectorant, carminative, rubefacient, emmenagogue (in large doses), decongestant, antispasmodic, antiseptic, nutritive

WHY I'M IN LOVE

It's generally agreed that the word *thyme* is derived from the Greek word *thumos*, meaning "courage." Don't underestimate the healing power of thyme. Sure, it's small—the leaves and flowers are not much bigger than a newborn's fingernail—but it packs a big punch. It is a strong antimicrobial agent, a skilled soother of respiratory conditions, an expert digestive aid, and a calming reliever of tension and anxiety.

WHAT IT DOES BEST

Thyme creeps and spreads through our bodies similar to the way it grows over the ground, blanketing us in healing warmth. You can find it in almost any kitchen, fresh or dried, and in practically every farmers market because of how crucial it is to our digestion. It's skilled at aiding an already healthy digestion system but can also enhance our appetites and relieve gas.

The volatile oils in thyme are what make it such a strong medicine. This powerful antimicrobial agent works well on the respiratory system. I like to make a facial steam with a bowl of hot water and a towel draped over my head. The hot steam alone does wonders for my skin and lungs but adding a handful of dried or a bunch of fresh thyme to the hot water simultaneously decongests and relieves chronic and acute respiratory conditions like laryngitis, sore throats, and a variety of wet coughs.

It's clear that thyme is good at moving things along to get us back to health, but it can also help us slow down to rest and reset. A mugful of warm thyme tea before bed can help ease mental and physical exhaustion, relieving the tension and anxiety that gets in the way of a good night's sleep. Since it's not a sedative it can be an appropriate tea to help you calm down and clear your mind in the middle of the day. Because it can turn up your internal temperature, I wouldn't choose to drink thyme tea before a big presentation, but it's great before a walk outside to clear your head on a cold day!

HOW IT GROWS

There are hundreds of species of thyme and all of them can be used interchangeably. Thyme is a low perennial evergreen shrub native to the Mediterranean. The leaves are oval and lance-shaped, bearing tiny purplish flowers that bloom from May to August. If you have thyme growing around your home or apartment, you can harvest enough medicine for you and probably a few of your friends by simply trimming the stalks multiple times from late spring through summer.

TO RECAP

Thyme has followed humans over many years to all corners of the world. In cooler months I always find thyme growing in the gardens of abandoned plots, even when most other cultivated plants have perished. Humans will always need to eat, and so long as we're faced with that task thyme makes the experience more enjoyable and more medicinal by easing the digestive process and warming us through.

Herbes de Provence Blend

Thyme is common in spice blends across cultures: you'll find it in jerk spice, za'atar, and herbes de Provence. It's easy enough to buy any of these blends at a market or grocery store, but it's more fun—and truly not that much effort—to make it at home, plus you can personalize it to your taste. I like this blend on any vegetables, fish, meat, and poultry, especially when a grill is involved. Depending on the season, I like to add dried citrus zest or tarragon, too. **Makes ½ cup.**

¼ cup dried thyme leaves

1 tablespoon dried chopped savory leaves

1 tablespoon dried chopped rosemary leaves

1 tablespoon dried and rubbed marjoram leaves

1 tablespoon dried and rubbed lavender flowers

Combine the ingredients in a mortar and pestle and gently muddle a few times. Stored in an airtight container out of direct sunlight, the blend will keep for up to 1 year. Be sure to gently crush the herbs as you sprinkle them onto whatever you're cooking.

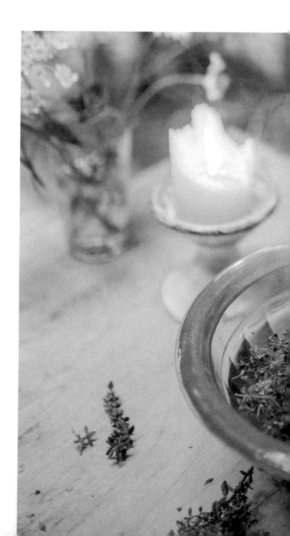

Thyme Facial Steam

When I was little and stuffed up or had a cough that wouldn't budge, my mom would steam up the bathroom and sit with me as we breathed in the hot, humid air. It was cozy and comforting. These days I'm not a squirmy toddler and so I can save water by making a mini version of this technique using a bowl and a towel. The power of thyme is an added bonus. An effective virus slayer and lung clearer, thyme helps loosen phlegm in the nose and respiratory track. Pro tip: keep a hanky nearby. **Makes 1 facial steam.**

1 bunch fresh thyme or a large handful dried thyme

Boil a kettle of water. While the water's boiling, gather a towel, hanky or tissues, and a heat-safe bowl. Put the thyme in the bowl, pour the water over, and cover your head and the bowl with the towel. Position your face over the bowl close enough to the steam so that you can breathe it in but not so close that you'll burn your face or nasal passages. Breathe slowly and deeply into your lungs, not your diaphragm. Your nose should start running in no time. Along with a clear nose, you'll get clear skin.

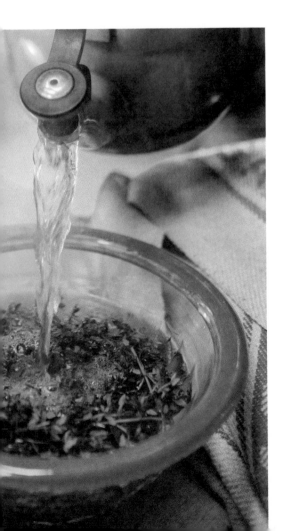

Violet

Viola odorata

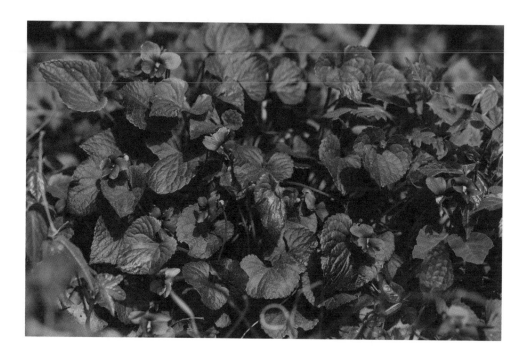

Reach for this when	You need a cooling demulcent, are working through a cough, experience inflammation
Sensation	Cooling, moistening
Flavors	Leaves: earthy Flowers: bright
Where it lives	Shady parts of the yard or park, especially under trees nestled among burdock, clovers, and dandelions
Gather this	Leaves and flowers (seeds and roots in the wrong amount can make you puke)
Super strengths	Alterative, demulcent, anti-inflammatory, cardiotonic, lymphagogue

WHY I'M IN LOVE

Violets are part of the spring welcoming committee! In the Northeast, March can sometimes feel unbearable and April desperate, but the beginning of May holds enough glimpses of hope to ease us into the new season.

For many of us, spring is a time of slow awakening and sometimes the pressure to be happy in spring elicits a rebellious retreat back indoors and under the covers. The emphasis on renewal and gratitude can feel pretty difficult. After a long winter, violet is a gentle introduction to spring. Violet is less pushy than other plants you might see around the same time, demanding less of us than say dandelion, whose bitterness beckons enthusiastically. Instead violet seems to say sweetly, "Congratulations, you made it."

WHAT IT DOES BEST

If you've heard the phrase "shrinking violet" you might be wondering how a flower that appears to be almost everywhere could acquire a modest, introverted association. It's perhaps only because mopey, British men walked around forests anthropomorphizing unassuming flora, likely with their own character traits. I personally find the violet to be a bold and bright presence in the world, a lush wreath of greenery and a gently beaming flower. The only shrinking violet might do is to the hard, hot places in your body. Swollen glands, irritated tonsils, bruises, or a temper about to burst are all places where violet can step in to nourish

and soothe. Violet is well suited for things that are brewing: the beginnings of an illness or stress where we feel hot and tight. If your impulse under anxiety is to clam up and sweat, violet can cool and relax.

Violet's soothing, nourishing actions make it well suited to dryness inside and on our bodies: constipation, skin, mouth, all the things involved in breathing, lymph nodes, eczema. When taken internally violet's moistening actions line our digestive system with slick mucilage all the way into our intestines. If you're backed up, violet's lubricating ability can help you get things moving. Instead of reaching for Smooth Move tea anytime you're having trouble pooping, just drink water infused with the benefits of violet leaf. In a few hours it'll slip right out of you, cramp free. What a relief.

If you love nettle infusion but find the effects drying on your already dry constitution, then consider violet leaf instead. It has a mild flavor, is mineral rich, and is high in vitamins A and C.

HOW IT GROWS

It's hard not to love a plant that is shaped like a heart. From violet's heart-shaped leaves spring a waving purple flag. The little flower head bends and bows over the damp, still-warming earth as we move into spring. There are hundreds of species of violet and once you learn how to identify this creeping perennial, you might see it everywhere. If you need help locating violets, follow the bees and butterflies to flowers of blue, purple, white, and yellow growing in the dappled light of cultivated earth. The simple toothed leaves grow in a basal arrangement and each flower is attached to a single stalk. Violets are hardly shy and hybridize easily (meaning they "hook up" across species), which makes it difficult to classify all of them. They're free-loving beautiful beings.

TO RECAP

Look for violet's deep green, heart-shaped leaves and purple flowers in May. As the weather warms toward the beginning of June the flowers go, but the leaves remain. Violet's flowers are charged with uplifting energy and its leaves offer a quiet, cool calm in the early buzz of spring. If you tend to shrink, stiffen, and get hot in the presence of change, whether sickness or seasonal, violet will provide the nourishment and moisture to work toward confidence and comfort.

> If you're subconsciously humming "All in the Golden Afternoon," dreaming you're some version of Alice in a trippy flower garden cozying up to the pansies, you're not far off track. You can distinguish pansies from violets by their petal arrangement: pansies have four petals facing up and one down (which makes that characteristic face of the cartoon flowers); violets have two petals up and three down.

Violet Syrup

This tastes like sweet spring in a bottle. It is delicious mixed into bubble water as a spring cocktail alternative, added to confectioner's sugar to make a glaze for baked goods, or just by the spoonful when you need to cultivate your inner garden. I like to use raw sugar, but if a loud purple is your thing, then go for granulated. (If you want to make a shelf-stable simple syrup, increase the sugar to achieve equal parts sugar and water.)
Makes 1½ cups.

1 cup water
½ cup raw or granulated sugar
1 cup fresh violet flowers
Juice of ½ lemon

Combine the water and sugar in a saucepan over medium-low heat. Heat, stirring occasionally, until the sugar dissolves—less than 5 minutes. Immediately add the violets, remove the pan from the heat, and cover the saucepan. When the syrup comes to room temperature, strain the flowers off the syrup and compost the plant material. Slowly add the lemon juice to the syrup until it turns a vibrant purple. Store the syrup in the refrigerator for up to a year.

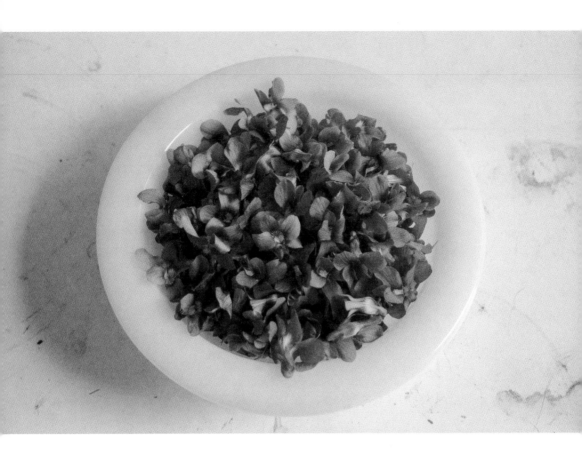

Lube Tea

This is a comforting, moistening, and mildly stimulating drink, especially skilled at moisturizing all of your insides that can make a big difference all through your body. This is a great tea for sexual health. Good, healthy sex starts on the inside. If you experience dryness from time to time, this tea is a cheap, natural remedy! **Makes 3½ cups.**

½ cup dried violet leaf

½ cup dried linden leaf and flower

¼ cup dried damiana leaves

¼ cup dried rose flowers

¼ cup dried tulsi leaves

1 tablespoon dried marshmallow root

Honey

Put all the dried herbs and root in a glass quart jar, cover with hot water, and let it steep 15 minutes. Add honey to taste. Place the jar in the refrigerator overnight and drink the next day.

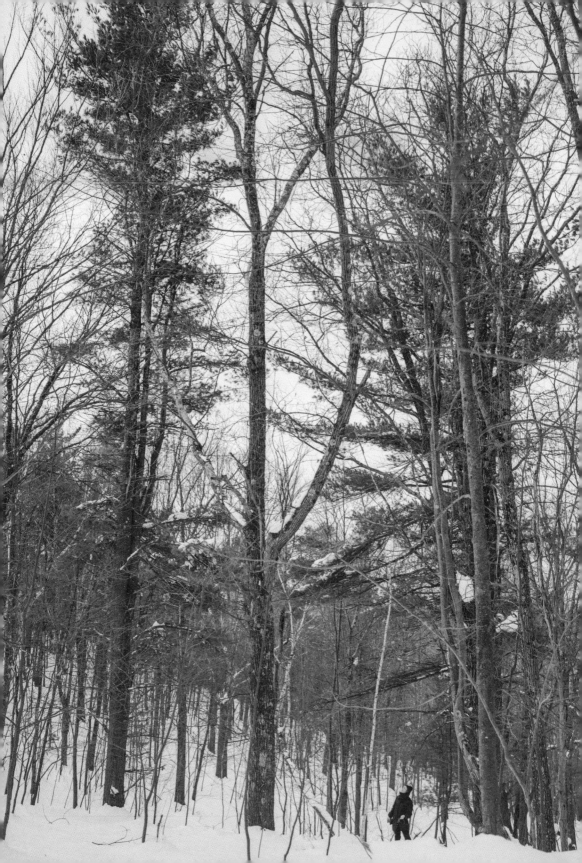

Acknowledgments

Though writing requires a lot of alone time, books are not written alone. I was able to write this book primarily because of the people I know and have known. Over thirty-five years that ends up being a lot of people! Thank you to the following individuals, without whom this book would have occupied the back burner of my mind and slowly turned to ash; because of you it has taken form.

While attending the University of Colorado Boulder, I lived in a blue house with a yard filled with wild things tended by the herbalist Brigitte Mars. She taught me about nettles: how to juice them, cook with them, and harvest them carefully enough to avoid their sting. I am thankful for her model of plant stewardship and eagerness to share and educate whenever the chance presented itself. From there I've been fortunate to study with herbalists and botanists from all over the United States. Thank you especially to my botany and herbal teachers: Robin Rose Bennett, Katja Swift, Ryn Midura, David Winston, Tammi Sweet, Wild Man Steve Brill, Nathaniel Whitmore, Richard Mandelbaum, Barbara Kurland, and Uli Lorimer. Eating for health and in care of the environment was not nearly as cool as it is today when I started to dabble in herbalism seventeen years ago and it certainly wasn't cool forty years ago. Thank you to my teachers and people like them for keeping herbal practice alive and for demonstrating what unwavering commitment to one's work looks like. Thank you for the excitement and enthusiasm present in your teachings and for sharing your invaluable experience with me and my fellow students.

I would also like to thank my professors at CU-Boulder: Patty Limerick, Mark Pittenger, Polly McLean, and Susan Kent, whose classes were the rare ones I attended. I think of them often, particularly their ability to help me navigate the triumphant, disappointing, and confusing circumstances of the past in an effort to forge a more thoughtful and hopeful future. Public school rules.

It was also in Colorado that I met Sara Bercholz at a bar on Pearl Street during an exceptionally beautiful snowstorm. Had I known she would publish my book nearly two decades later I think I would have puked, then excused myself from the table and our friendship. Thankfully, we had no idea, and over the years we've nourished a relationship that now includes siblings, partners, children, and more friends. I can't think of anyone else with whom I'd want to make a book. I am so proud of what she's accomplished with Roost and so honored to be a part of it.

Where would I be if not for the amazing team of editors at Roost? Juree Sondker taught me everything that I now know about writing a book. And she made it fun! Thank you for your patience, guidance, and firm commitment to deadlines. Thank you for taking my wild ideas seriously and helping me figure out how to get them into the world. Also, thank you to Audra Figgins, Mollie Firestone, and Jill Rogers for their attention, thoughtful commentary, and thorough editing.

A big and special thank you to my pal and photographer for this book Lawrence Braun. What better way to spend a year than outside shooting plants with one of your best pals? There were times when I just could not imagine this book ever getting done, and inevitably the balm was to go outside together. For me, our explorations and meanderings were as essential to my health as eating well and sleeping enough. Thank you also to his family, Jessica and Forest, for their generosity of time.

The food media world is a small and excellent group of talented, heartful, and dedicated people. They have indulged my personal projects, taught me everything I know about styling for photography, and become dear friends. Thanks to Samantha Bolton and Joe Lingeman, who I work with every day. They are fantastic colleagues and their input was invaluable as I worked to write and shoot this book. To the food stylists who taught me everything I know, thank you for taking me under your wing: Maggie Ruggiero, Rebecca Jurkevich, Anne Disrude, Vivian Lui, and last but certainly not least Cyd McDowell. If it weren't for Cyd this book wouldn't have nearly as many beautiful photographs as it does. Thank you for feeding me, picking me up from the train station, letting me shoot in your house and garden, giving me books to read, asking me questions, swimming in the lake with me, staying up late to process and dream, and for being my cheerleader. Cyd, I am eternally grateful for your commitment to this book, our friendship, and for all you've taught me.

A big thank you to all of my friends who scraped me off the floor, propped me in a seated position and maintained that I could do this. Thank you for tolerating an extreme spike in my hermetic proclivities (I can't believe it was even possible to get more extreme!) while I conceived of, wrote, shot, and edited this book. And I owe you all an apology for invitations declined and long stretches of radio silence: I am grateful that I still have you on the other side. Because I have no shame and am unbearably sentimental, I am going to list all of you. Ted Kerr, Mars Singer, Max Freeman, and Scott Lyman for being my Team, believing in me, and insisting I get out of my apartment even if it was just to work more in a different location. Sarah Lowe for so much, but especially for your wisdom offered at The Magician. Paul Dana and Sue Li for helping me pick allelopathic plants in Prospect Park. Brittany Ducham for navigating the highs and lows of the publishing process. Dude, thanks for coming on this wild ride. Clayton Lewis for being my nerdiest herb pal and my first partner in formal training. Nat Wilkin for uplifting trans-oceanic skypes. Brooke Baxter Bailey and Thimali Kodikara for always being in my heart and life no matter where we are. William Purcell for always sending sweet vibes. Kate Heilmann Bo for braving the snow and being the driving force behind my most memorable encounter with nettles. Zak Rosen and Shira Heisler for boldly demonstrating their affection for me. Sharon Katzoff for always leaving her door open to me. Gabriela Alvarez and Shira Moss for letting me into their hearts and minds; you were both instrumental to my thinking and moving through this process. My dear pals, Mo Connolly and Nicole Lewis, thank you for demonstrating what a bottomless lake of love looks like. Not to brag, but I am lucky to have many people who love me and whom I love.

Thank you to my mum, my Aunt Monique, and my sister. Thank you, Mum and Monique, who taught me that you don't have to be unbearably "outdoorsy" to prove that you love the outdoors, and who modeled that the simplest way to make a home more livable is to open your windows and doors to the outside and welcome the wild in no matter where you are. Better yet, just host every cocktail hour and meal outside. And to my sister, Liza, who is endlessly curious and bravely open to the wonders of our earth.

Working a full-time job in a wonderfully hectic city meant that most of this book was written whenever (and wherever) it could be: on my phone, laptop, and scraps of paper while walking to and riding the beautiful NYC subway, sitting in the back of friend's cars (thanks Shuls!), on Amtrak and Metro-North, and riding in airplanes. For that, I would like to thank the MTA, the Interstate Highway System, and major airline carriers.

I would be remiss not to acknowledge the people I have never met. I am thankful for herbalists, activists, healers, and members of communities that have been marginalized who keep these practices alive in spaces and times that refused to see them or acknowledge their past and ongoing contributions. I am thinking here of indigenous communities, people of color, women, people of non-binary gender, people with disabilities and all the people who live at the intersection of the aforementioned ways of being alive—of being human. Who, throughout history, relied on the land and each other to ensure that their people would survive. I also want to acknowledge that much of what we know about certain plants and healing practices was stolen or learned from indigenous and enslaved people whose right to live freely and healthfully in the world was violently taken from them.

Lastly, I am grateful for the determination of the natural world: to the plants and animals that refuse to give in to the conditions of the Anthropocene and in so doing remind us that we all have a place and a right to a healthful life on earth. The responsibility to ensure that rests in each of us.

Resources

Websites

BOTANY AND FIELD RELATED REFERENCE

United Plant Savers: unitedplantsavers.org

Missouri Botanical Garden: missouribotanicalgarden.org

Kew Gardens: kew.org

Go Botany–Northeast: gobotany.nativeplanttrust.org

USDA Plants: plants.sc.egov.usda.gov

MATERIA MEDICA

Nicholas Culpepper: complete-herbal.com

Herb Mentor: learningherbs.com

Maude Grieve: botanical.com

Books

HERBALISM

Richo Cech, *Making Plant Medicines*

Rosalee de la Forêt, *Alchemy of Herbs: Transform Everyday Ingredients into Foods and Remedies That Heal*

James Green, *The Herbal Medicine-Maker's Handbook: A Home Manual*

Maude Grieve, *A Modern Herbal: The Complete Edition*

David Hoffman, *Medical Herbalism: The Science and Practice of Herbal Medicine*

Henriette Kress, *Practical Herbs*

Guido Masé, *The Wild Medicine Solution: Healing with Aromatic, Bitter, and Tonic Plants*

Matthew Wood, *The Earthwise Herbal, Volume I: A Complete Guide to Old World Medicinal Plants*

Matthew Wood, *The Earthwise Herbal, Volume II: A Complete Guide to New World Medicinal Plants*

David Winston and Steven Maimes, *Adaptogens: Herbs for Strength, Stamina, and Stress Relief*

BOTANY AND FIELD GUIDES

Brian Capon, *Botany for Gardeners*

Thomas Elpel, *Botany in a Day: The Patterns Method of Plant Identification*

Roger Tory Peterson and Margaret McKenny, *A Peterson Field Guide to Wildflowers: Northeastern and North-Central North America*

Wendy B. Zomlefer, *Guide to Flowering Plant Families*

Where to Buy

HERBS

Sourcing locally is preferred, but not all of us can do that! Fortunately you can order from small, local farms with relative ease.

Black Locust Gardens—Michigan: blacklocustgardens.com

Freedom Food Farm—Massachusetts: freedomfoodfarm.com

Friends of the Trees—Pacific Northwest: friendsofthetrees.net

Frontier Herbs—Iowa: frontiercoop.com

Gentle Harmony Farm—North Carolina: gentleharmonyfarm.com

Healing Spirits Herb Farm—New York: healingspiritsherbfarm.com

Herban Ayurveda—Minnesota: herbanayurveda.com

Mountain Rose Herbs—Pacific Northwest: mountainroseherbs.com

Pacific Botanicals—Oregon: pacificbotanicals.com

Sawmill Herb Farm—Massachusetts: sawmillherbfarm.com

Zack Woods Farm—Vermont: zackwoodsherbs.com

SEAWEEDS

Maine Seaweed LLC—Maine: theseaweedman.com

Island Herbs—Washington: ryandrum.com

Atlantic Holdfast—Maine: holdfastseaweed.com

MEDICINE-MAKING SUPPLIES, TINS, BOSTON ROUND BOTTLES, ETC.

Berlin Packaging: berlinpackaging.com

CANNING JARS

Fresh Preserving: freshpreserving.com

Bibliography

Bergner, Paul. "Herbs and Insulin Resistance." *Medical Herbalism: A Journal for the Clinical Practitioner* 13, no. 2 (Winter 2002–2003): 1–9.

———. *The Healing Power of Garlic.* California: Prima Publishing, 1996.

Culpepper, Nicholas. *Complete Herbal.* London: Foulsham, 1880.

De La Forêt, Rosalee. *Alchemy of Herbs: Transform Everyday Ingredients into Foods and Remedies That Heal.* New York: Hay House, 2017.

Elpel, Thomas J. *Botany in a Day: The Patterns Method of Plant Identification.* 5th ed. Pony, MT: Hops Press, 2004.

Francis, Deborah. "Nourishing the Nerves." *Medical Herbalism: A Journal for the Clinical Practitioner,* 12, no. 1 (January 2001): 1, 6–7.

Gladstar, Rosemary. *Medicinal Herbs: A Beginner's Guide.* North Adams, MA: Storey Publishing, 2012

Green, James. *The Herbal Medicine Maker's Handbook: A Home Manual.* New York: Crossing Press, 2000.

Grieve, Maude. *A Modern Herbal.* New York: Dover Publications, Inc., 1971.

Guido, Masé. *The Wild Medicine Solution: Healing with Aromatic, Bitter, and Tonic Plants.* Rochester, VT: Healing Arts Press, 2013.

Hoffman, David. *The Holistic Herbal.* Rochester, VT: The Findhorn Press. 1983.

Hoffman, David. *Medical Herbalism: The Science and Practice of Herbal Medicine.* 1st ed. Rochester, VT: Healing Arts Press, 2003.

Kress, Henriette. *Practical Herbs.* Sweden: Yrtit ja yrttiterapia Henriette Kress, 2013.

Lindlahr, Henry. *Nature Cure.* CreateSpace, 2013.

Mabey, Richard. *The New Age Herbalist.* London: Gaia Books, 1988.

Remington, Joseph, and Horatio Wood. 20th ed. *The Dispensatory of the United States of America.* Philadelphia, PA: Lippincott Company, 1918.

Winston, David and Maimes, Steven. *Adaptogens: Herbs for Strength, Stamina, and Stress Relief.* Rochester, VT: Healing Arts Press, 2007.

Wood, Matthew. *The Book of Herbal Wisdom: Using Plants as Medicine.* Berkeley, CA: North Atlantic Books, 1997.

———. *The Practice of Traditional Western Herbalism: Basic Doctrine, Energetics, and Classification.* Berkeley, CA: North Atlantic Books, 2004.

———. *The Earthwise Herbal, Volume I: A Complete Guide to Old World Medicinal Plants.* Berkeley, CA: North Atlantic Books, 2008.

———. *The Earthwise Herbal, Volume II: A Complete Guide to New World Medicinal Plants.* Berkeley, CA: North Atlantic Books, 2008.

Young, Paul. *The Botany Coloring Book.* New York: Harper Perennial, 1982.

Index

About the Author

Christine Buckley is a community-based herbalist, professional cook, and visual artist. Her writing has appeared in *Well + Good*, Kitchn, and *Healthyish*, and she has displayed work at the Honolulu Biennial and MoMA Studios. She has cooked in some of New York's best restaurants and most recently worked as a food stylist. She studied herbalism at the Commonwealth Center for Holistic Herbalism and the Center for Herbal Studies. This is her first book.